RETINA

Allen C. Ho, MD

Associate Professor of Ophthalmology
Thomas Jefferson University
Retina Service
Wills Eye Hospital
Philadelphia, Pennsylvania

Franco M. Recchia, MD

Fellow
Vitreoretinal Surgery
Associated Retinal Consultants, PC
William Beaumont Hospital
Royal Oak, Michigan

Gary C. Brown, MD

Professor of Ophthalmology
Thomas Jefferson University
Retina Service
Wills Eye Hospital
Philadelphia, Pennsylvania

Carl D. Regillo, MD

Associate Professor of Ophthalmology
Thomas Jefferson University
Retina Service
Wills Eye Hospital
Philadelphia, Pennsylvania

J. Arch McNamara, MD

Assistant Professor of Ophthalmology
Thomas Jefferson University
Retina Service
Wills Eye Hospital
Philadelphia, Pennsylvania

James F. Vander, MD

Associate Professor of Ophthalmology
Thomas Jefferson University
Retina Service
Wills Eye Hospital
Philadelphia, Pennsylvania

McGraw-Hill
MEDICAL PUBLISHING DIVISION

New York   Chicago   San Francisco   Lisbon   London
Madrid   Mexico City   Milan   New Delhi   San Juan   Seoul
Singapore   Sydney   Toronto

Retina: Color Atlas & Synopsis of Clinical Ophthalmology

Copyright © 2003 by The **McGraw-Hill** Companies, Inc. All rights reserved. Printed in Spain. Except as permitted under the United States Copyright Act of 1976, no part of this publication may be reproduced or distributed in any form or by any means, or stored in a data base or retrieval system, without the prior written permission of the publisher.

1234567890   IMP/IMP   098765432

ISBN 0-07-137596-1

This book was set in Times Roman by TechBooks.
The editors were Darlene Cooke, Susan Noujaim, and Karen Davis.
The production supervisor was Catherine Saggese.
The book designer was Marsha Cohen.
The cover designer was Mary Belibasakis.
The index was prepared by Editorial Services, Maria Coughlin.
Cayfosa-Quebecor, Barcelona, was printer and binder.

This book is printed on acid-free paper.

NOTICE

Medicine is an ever-changing science. As new research and clinical experience broaden our knowledge, changes in treatment and drug therapy are required. The authors and the publisher of this work have checked with sources believed to be reliable in their efforts to provide information that is complete and generally in accord with the standards accepted at the time of publication. However, in view of the possibility of human error or changes in medical sciences, neither the authors nor the publisher nor any other party who has been involved in the preparation or publication of this work warrants that the information contained herein is in every respect accurate or complete, and they disclaim all responsibility for any errors or omissions or for the results obtained from use of the information contained in this work. Readers are encouraged to confirm the information contained herein with other sources. For example and in particular, readers are advised to check the product information sheet included in the package of each drug they plan to administer to be certain that the information contained in this work is accurate and that changes have not been made in the recommended dose or in the contraindications for administration. This recommendation is of particular importance in connection with new or infrequently used drugs.

Library of Congress Cataloging-in-Publication Data

Retina: Color atlas & synopsis of clinical ophthalmology / Allen Ho ... [et al.].
    p.;   cm.—(Color atlas & synopsis of clinical ophthalmology series)
    Includes bibliographical references and index.
    ISBN 0-07-137596-1
    1. Retina—Diseases—Atlases. 2. Retina—Diseases—Handbooks, manuals, etc.   I. Ho, Allen.
II. Series.
    [DNLM: 1. Retinal Diseases—Atlases.   WW 17 R438 2003]
RE551 .R447   2003
617.7'35—dc21

2002075354

COLOR ATLAS &

SYNOPSIS OF

CLINICAL

OPHTHALMOLOGY

WILLS EYE HOSPITAL

RETINA

COLOR ATLAS AND SYNOPSIS OF CLINICAL OPHTHALMOLOGY SERIES

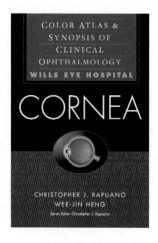

CORNEA
Christopher J. Rapuano, MD
Wee-Jin Heng, MD
0-07-137589-9

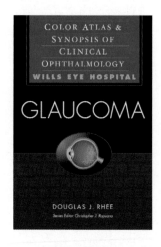

GLAUCOMA
Douglas J. Rhee, MD
0-07-137597-X

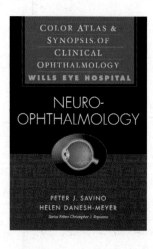

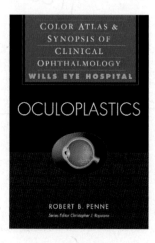

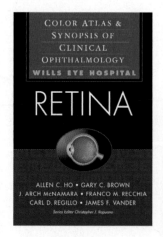

NEUROOPHTHALMOLOGY
Peter J. Savino, MD
Helen Danesh-Meyer, MD
0-07-137595-3

OCULOPLASTICS
Robert B. Penne, MD
0-07-137594-5

RETINA
Allen C. Ho, MD
Gary C. Brown, MD
J. Arch McNamara, MD
Franco M. Recchia, MD
Carl D. Regillo, MD
James F. Vander, MD
0-07-137596-1

CONTENTS

Chapter 5

Chapter 6

RETINAL DEGENERATIONS AND DYSTROPHIES   **142**
Mithlesh Sharma and Allen C. Ho

Chapter 7

RETINAL AND CHOROIDAL TUMORS   **178**
Franco M. Recchia

Chapter 8

CONGENITAL AND PEDIATRIC RETINAL DISEASES   **206**
J. Arch McNamara

Chapter 9

TRAUMATIC AND TOXIC RETINOPATHIES 228
J. Luigi Borrillo, and Carl D. Regillo

Chapter 10

PERIPHERAL RETINAL DISEASE 258
James F. Vander

CONTRIBUTORS

J.Luigi Borrillo, MD

Fellow
Retina Service
Wills Eye Hospital
Philadelphia, Pennsylvania

Gary C. Brown, MD

Professor of Ophthalmology
Thomas Jefferson University
Retina Service
Wills Eye Hospital
Philadelphia, Pennsylvania

Allen C. Ho, MD

Associate Professor of Ophthalmology
Thomas Jefferson University
Retina Service
Wills Eye Hospital
Philadelphia, Pennsylvania

J. Arch McNamara, MD

Assistant Professor of Ophthalmology
Thomas Jefferson University
Retina Service
Wills Eye Hospital
Philadelphia, Pennsylvania

Franco M. Recchia, MD

Fellow
Vitreoretinal Surgery
Associated Retinal Consultants, PC
William Beaumont Hospital
Royal Oak, Michigan

Carl D. Regillo, MD

Associate Professor of Ophthalmology
Thomas Jefferson University
Retina Service
Wills Eye Hospital
Philadelphia, Pennsylvania

Mithlesh Sharma, MD

Retina Fellow
Eye and Ear Intirmary
University of Illinois at Chicago
Chicago, Illinois

Magdalena F. Shuler, MD

Fellow
Retina Service
Wills Eye Hospital
Philadelphia, Pennsylvania

James F. Vander, MD

Associate Professor of Ophthalmology
Thomas Jefferson University
Retina Service
Wills Eye Hospital
Philadelphia, Pennsylvania

Imaging Consultants

Jay Klancnik, MD

Henry C. Lee, MD

ABOUT THE SERIES

The beauty of the atlas/synopsis concept is the powerful combination of illustrative photographs and a summary approach to the text. Ophthalmology is a very visual discipline which lends itself nicely to clinical photographs. While the five ophthalmic subspecialties in this series, Cornea, Retina, Glaucoma, Oculoplastics, and Neuroophthalmology, employ varying levels of visual recognition, a relatively standard format for the text is used for all volumes.

The goal of the series is to provide an up-to-date clinical overview of the major areas of ophthalmology for students, residents, and practitioners in all the healthcare professions. The abundance of large, excellent quality photographs and concise, outline-form text will help achieve that objective.

Christopher J. Rapuano, MD.
Series Editor

PREFACE

Vitreoretinal disease is a privileged visual discipline. There are significant barriers to its study beyond the constricted pupil. Ophthalmology trainees first acquire the observational skills and facility with diagnostic instrumentation such as the slit lamp biomicroscope and the indirect ophthalmoscope to begin to explore diseases that affect the posterior segment of the eye. It takes clinical experience to discern normal variation from significant pathology. Unfortunately, most nonophthalmic physicians are limited to facility with the direct ophthalmoscope that only affords a keyhole view of the back of the eye. We are privileged to be lifelong students, practitioners, clinical researchers and teachers of this aspect of the eye here at Wills Eye Hospital.

When we were asked to create a concise color atlas and synopsis of vitreoretinal disease we knew our challenges would be to be concise and to be selective since there is great richness of clinical detail, both visually and with words. Our aim was to balance the breadth of the subject material with enough focused detail to provide the framework of our thinking regarding important clinical signs, associated clinical signs, differential diagnosis, diagnostic evaluation, and prognosis and management of hundreds of vitreoretinal conditions. We want this to be a "go to" field manual but realize that it cannot be an encyclopedic reference.

The images of this color atlas and synopsis include over 300 color images and over 100 black and white images, typically fluorescein angiographic images. Each was digitized from an original photographic slide as a high resolution RGB image, at least 1500 pixels by 1200 pixels. Our goals were to present the images in their highest quality native colors and contrasts, to limit photographic artifact, and to highlight certain clinical features of the images with annotations or image insets. Every effort was made to maintain the integrity of the original photographs, with frequent reference to the original source. Image enhancement was reserved only for the selected image insets of this work, in cases where we felt particular features could be better illustrated with digital manipulation. We often magnified (though at no time was interpolation used to create new pixels) the insets, made them grayscale, and increased the contrast for the ease of the reader.

Ultimately, our intent is to present this color atlas and synopsis as an aid to the diagnosis and management of vitreoretinal diseases in the care of patients and as a resource for students of these conditions.

COLOR ATLAS &
SYNOPSIS OF
CLINICAL
OPHTHALMOLOGY

WILLS EYE HOSPITAL

RETINA

Chapter 1

AGE-RELATED MACULAR DEGENERATION

Allen C. Ho, MD

Age-related macular degeneration (AMD) describes a common degenerative condition of the retina that may affect central vision. By definition, it occurs in individuals 50 years and older and is more prevalent with increasing age. Population-based surveys in the Western world vary but estimate the prevalence of AMD to be approximately 10% to 35% in individuals over the age of 50 years. Age-related macular degeneration is divided into "dry" or nonexudative AMD and "wet" or exudative AMD.

DRY OR NONEXUDATIVE AGE-RELATED MACULAR DEGENERATION

Definition

Drusen are the clinical hallmark of dry AMD. They are subretinal pigment epithelial deposits between the basement membrane of the retinal pigment epithelium (RPE) and Bruch's membrane (Figures 1-1 and 1-2). Multiple types of drusen have been described, including large drusen (greater than 64 μm); small drusen (63 μm or smaller); calcified drusen, which are yellow and glistening; and basal laminar drusen, which are small round diffuse drusen that are more apparent on fluorescein angiography than on clinical fundus examination (Figure 1-3).

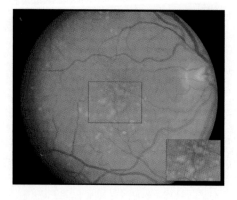

Figure 1-1 Large drusen *Fundus photograph demonstrating predominantly large drusen, some of which are confluent* (inset). *Visual acuity was 20/25.*

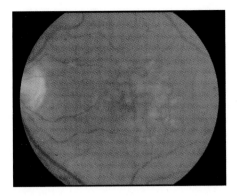

Figure 1-2 Confluent drusen *Fundus photograph demonstrating multiple large, predominantly confluent drusen. Confluence is greatest temporal to the fovea. Confluent drusen are a risk factor for exudative age-related macular degeneration (AMD).*

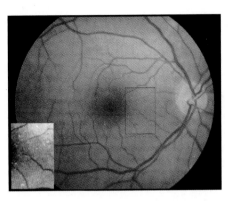

Figure 1-3 Basal laminar drusen
Fundus photograph demonstrating multiple small, round, diffuse drusen (inset) with large areas of confluence in the posterior pole and midperipheral retina. Basal laminar drusen may be more apparent with fluorescein angiography than clinically.

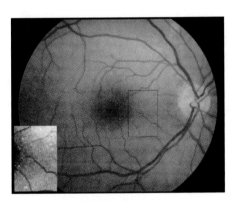

Figure 1-4 Hard drusen *Hard drusen (inset) are small (63 μm or smaller) and are not a risk factor for more advanced forms of AMD.*

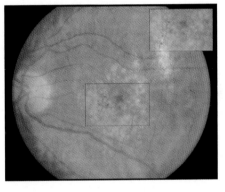

Figure 1-5 Focal hyperpigmentation
Fundus photograph showing multiple drusen with retinal pigment epithelial alterations (inset). Focal hyperpigmentation is noted in the fovea and just nasal to the fovea. Focal hyperpigmentation is a risk factor for more advanced forms of AMD associated with vision loss.

Multiple large drusen are representative of a diffuse thickening of Bruch's membrane. Large drusen, also known as soft drusen, are a risk factor for more advanced AMD and vision loss. Small (also known as hard) drusen alone do not increase the risk for more advanced forms of AMD (Figure 1-4).

Retinal pigment epithelial abnormalities, including nongeographic atrophy, focal hyperpigmentation, and frank geographic atrophy, are also common fundus features of dry AMD (Figure 1-5). Granularity of the RPE may be an early feature of retinal pigment epithelial disturbance due to AMD.

This may progress to areas of nongeographic atrophy (Figure 1-6A,B) in which there is loss of pigment of the RPE, but this is not discrete, and underlying choroidal vessels are not apparent. Geographic atrophy comprises discrete loss of RPE in a so-called cookie-cutter fashion with a minimal diameter of 250 μm associated with underlying loss of choroidal stromal pigment and clearly visible underlying larger choroidal vessels (Figure 1-7).

Epidemiology and Etiology

Drusen are seen increasingly with advancing age and typically are present in the sixth decade of life or later. Population-based studies estimate approximately 10% prevalence of early AMD (drusen) in the fifth decade of life, increasing to 35% in the seventh decade. Drusen may be seen in younger patients and may be heritable in these cases. The precise source of drusen material is not completely

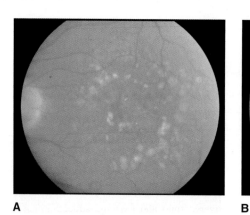 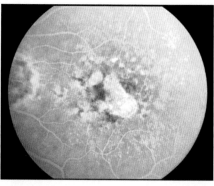

A   **B**

Figure 1-6A,B Nongeographic atrophy *A. Multiple large drusen are noted and there are areas of retinal pigment epithelial alterations. Surrounding the fovea superiorly and temporally are two areas of nongeographic atrophy. There is thinning of the retinal pigment epithelium (RPE), but the borders are not discrete around the entire lesion and the underlying larger choroidal vessels are not visible at this time. B. Fluorescein angiogram demonstrating transmission hyperfluorescence in nongeographic atrophy. Later images do not demonstrate leakage.*

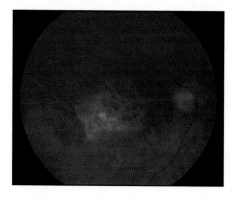

Figure 1-7 End-stage geographic atrophy *Large geographic atrophy involving the fovea. Note the visibility of the underlying larger choroidal vessels. Visual acuity was counting fingers.*

CHAPTER 1. AGE-RELATED MACULAR DEGENERATION

understood, but they are thought to represent degenerative products of retinal pigment epithelial cells; they are composed of lipids and glycoproteins, and may be mineralized. Retinal pigment epithelial alterations are seen increasingly with age and are common in the seventh, eighth, and ninth decades of life.

Pathology

Transmission electron microscopy of eyes with drusen and dry AMD shows two types of deposits:

Basal laminar deposits consist of wide-spaced collagen localized between the retinal pigment epithelial plasma membrane and the retinal pigment epithelial basement membrane.

Basal linear deposits consist of lipid-rich material external to the basement membrane of the RPE in the inner collagenous zone of Bruch's membrane.

History

Patients with drusen may be visually asymptomatic. Patients with multiple drusen and associated retinal pigment epithelial abnormalities including granularity of the RPE, atrophy of the RPE, or focal hyperpigmentation will often note fluctuating vision, including central blurring. They typically will describe a need for increased light intensity in order to read and have difficulty adapting between different lighting. Patients with dry AMD and without evidence of geographic atrophy of the RPE or exudative AMD typically have good central vision between 20/20 and 20/60.

Clinical and Fluorescein Angiographic Signs

Fundus biomicroscopy shows subretinal pale yellow deposits that may vary in size from greater than 64 μm (large drusen) to small or hard drusen (63 μm or smaller) in diameter. Calcific drusen have a glistening appearance, and most patients with AMD have a mixture of clinical drusen types. Large drusen will often become confluent into larger drusenoid pigment epithelial detachments. Drusen should be considered fluid and dynamic structures that can appear or resolve over time (Figure 1-8A,B).

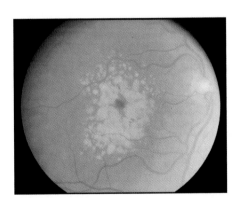

Figure 1-8A Drusenoid pigment epithelial detachment *Right eye of a patient showing large confluent drusen in a drusenoid pigment epithelial detachment configuration. There is focal hyperpigmentation centered on the fovea. Visual acuity was 20/40.*

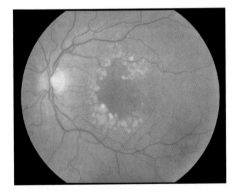

Figure 1-8B Drusenoid pigment epithelial detachment, resolved *Left eye of the same patient as Figure 1-8A showing spontaneous resolution of a drusenoid pigment epithelial detachment with a residual rim of confluent large drusen. Visual acuity was 20/30.*

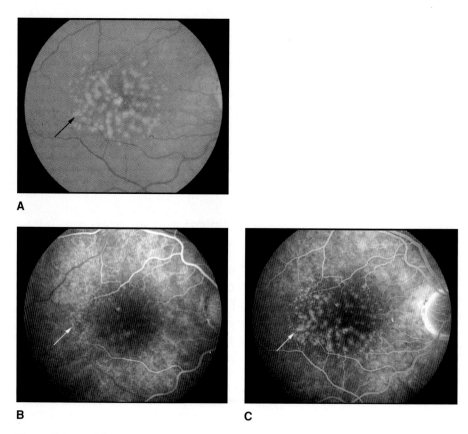

Figure 1-9   Multiple large drusen and confluent drusen   *A. Drusen may spontaneously regress and progress to areas of right pigment epithelial atrophy* (arrow). *There is loss of foveal pigment from spontaneous resolution of drusen.* ***B.*** *Early-phase fluorescein angiogram demonstrating mild relative hypofluorescence corresponding to drusen* (arrow). ***C.*** *Recirculation phase of fluorescein angiogram showing staining of drusen as discrete areas of hyperfluorescence* (arrow).

An irregular granular appearance to the RPE is often seen in association with drusen. Areas of nongeographic atrophy or frank geographic atrophy are often appreciated after the spontaneous resolution of drusen and, in particular, drusenoid pigment epithelial detachments. Intraretinal pigment clumps or focal hyperpigmentation represents advanced retinal pigment epithelial degeneration as well.

Fluorescein angiography typically demonstrates a patchy hyper- and hypofluorescence without leakage of dye. Drusen may show early or late hyperfluorescence, depending on the integrity of the overlying RPE and the histochemistry of the drusen themselves. Large soft drusen typically show early hypofluorescence and late hyperfluorescence (Figure 1-9A–C). This angiographic pattern is inconsistent, how-

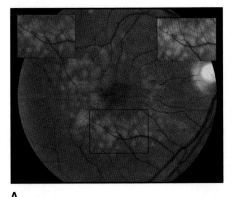

A

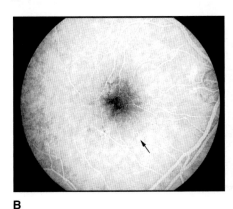

B

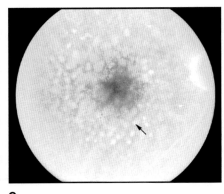

C

Figure 1-10 Multiple large drusen *A. Multiple large confluent drusen* (insets). *Visual acuity was 20/25.* ***B.** Fluorescein angiogram showing early hyperfluorescence of the large drusen* (arrow). ***C.** Late fluorescein angiogram showing drusen staining but no evidence of choroidal neovascularization (CNV,* arrow).

ever, because some drusen, even those that are large, will show earlier hyperfluorescence (Figure 1-10A–C). Geographic atrophy shows discrete hyperfluorescence with stable boundaries throughout the angiogram (Figure 1-11A–D).

Associated Clinical Signs

When drusen are noted in patients over the age of 50, other features of AMD are often observed, including granularity and atrophy of the RPE. Drusen that are associated with subretinal fluid, hemorrhage, or lipid exudation due to choroidal neovascularization are characteristic of exudative AMD.

Differential Diagnosis

Drusen are subretinal and should be distinguished from intraretinal processes such as intraretinal lipid, retinal emboli, and cotton-wool spots. The borders of drusen may be more distinct in smaller hard drusen and less distinct with large drusen.

Other yellow macular lesions can be included in the differential diagnosis of drusen. Pattern dystrophy, Best's dystrophy, multifocal Best's disease, and adult foveal macular dystrophy all can be confused with typical drusen of AMD (Table 1-1).

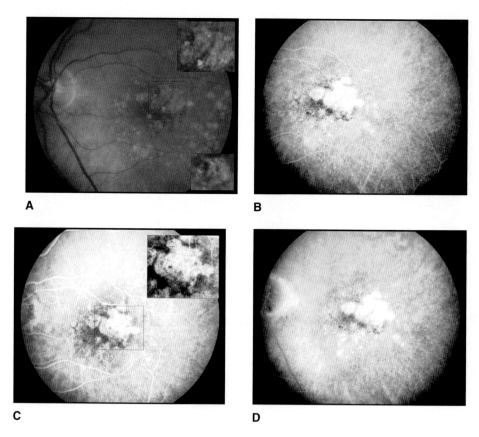

Figure 1-11 Atrophic AMD *A. Color fundus photograph demonstrating atrophic AMD. Multiple large and medium-sized drusen are noted, and an area of geographic atrophy is noted just superior to the fovea* (inset upper right). *The borders are discrete, and the larger underlying choroidal vessels are visible. Areas of focal hyperpigmentation are noted as well* (inset lower right). *B. Early-phase fluorescein angiogram demonstrating transmission hyperfluorescence in the area of geographic atrophy. C. Recirculation phase photograph shows hyperfluorescence in the area of geographic atrophy but no evidence of leakage* (inset). *D. Late-phase fluorescein angiogram showing some fading of the choroidal fluorescence and staining hyperfluorescence in the region of geographic atrophy.*

TABLE 1-1 DRUSEN DIFFERENTIAL DIAGNOSIS

Pattern dystrophy	Presents in younger patients; lesions show geographic shape
Best's disease	Round or oval lesions may show different stages
Adult foveomacular dystrophy	Yellowish green subfoveal lesion; may simulate choroidal neovascularization on fluorescein angiography

TABLE 1-2 RISK OF CHOROIDAL NEOVASCULARIZATION (CNV) FOR EYES WITH DRUSEN (FELLOW EYE WITH EXUDATIVE CNV)

Overall estimate is 10% of patients per year with unilateral drusen will develop CNV. The Macular Photocoagulation Study Group has established risk factors that increase the risk of CNV:

Multiple large drusen
Focal hyperpigmentation
Hypertension
Smoking

Diagnostic Evaluation

Patients with a sudden change in vision or new blur or distortion of central vision may be evaluated with fluorescein angiography to rule out exudative AMD. Careful fundus biomicroscopy is important to rule out subtle signs of exudative AMD (Table 1-2).

Prognosis and Management

Patients with drusen are counseled that they have the dry form of AMD and that the majority of patients with drusen will not develop vision loss due to more advanced forms of AMD (exudative AMD and choroidal neovascularization [CNV] or geographic atrophy). Patients with multiple large drusen are at a higher risk of developing CNV, particularly if the fellow eye has previously developed exudative AMD. The 5-year risk of developing CNV in fellow eyes of patients with exudative AMD ranges between 40% and 85%. Management includes counseling regarding the importance of monitoring central vision in each eye with a test object such as the Amsler grid (Figure 1-12).

Information from the Age-Related Eye Disease Study demonstrates that micronutrient and antioxidant supplementation (vitamin C, 500 mg; vitamin E, 400 IU; beta carotene, 15 mg; zinc, 80 mg as zinc oxide; and copper, 2 mg as cupric oxide) can effect a modest but definite reduction in clinical progression of AMD and moderate visual loss in patients with dry AMD and at least one large druse of 125 μm or larger. Data were not significant for patients with mild or borderline dry AMD (multiple small drusen or nonextensive intermediate drusen of 63 to 124 μm, pigment abnormalities, or any combination of these).

Patients with focal hyperpigmentation have a higher risk of developing more advanced forms of AMD associated with vision loss and, in particular, CNV. Some believe that this clinical feature may represent a sign of early, ill-defined CNV in many cases. If there is a suspicion of early exudative AMD, then fluorescein angiography may be performed. Because early retinal pigment epithelial abnormalities and granularity of the RPE may lead to nongeographic atrophy and frank geographic atrophy, they may be harbingers of vision loss.

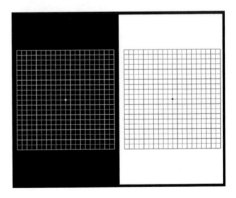

Figure 1-12 Amsler grids *Patients are instructed to monitor their central vision one eye at a time. Distortion, blurriness, or missing areas should prompt evaluation.*

EXUDATIVE AGE-RELATED MACULAR DEGENERATION

Definition

Exudative AMD is characterized by subretinal or subretinal pigment epithelial leakage, hemorrhage, or lipid exudation. Choroidal neovascularization is the abnormal growth of new choroidal vessels into the subretinal space through defects in Bruch's membrane. In AMD, CNV may be intertwined in Bruch's membrane and the retinal pigment epithelium. Younger patients (non-AMD) who develop CNV typically develop this vascularization in the subretinal space alone. Pigment epithelial detachment describes a blister-like elevation of the retinal pigment epithelium and is another form of exudative AMD. Pigment epithelial detachments may be vascularized (fibrovascular pigment epithelial detachment) or may be purely serous and not associated with CNV. Disciform scarring is a final common pathway of CNV and pigment epithelial detachment in which there is progressive fibrosis and loss of macular photoreceptor function (Figure 1-13).

Although the prevalence of the exudative form of AMD is low (approximately 10% of all patients with AMD), this form of late AMD accounts for the majority of legally blind patients with AMD (90%). The incidence of exudative AMD is on the rise, with an estimated 200,000 individuals experiencing severe central loss of vision due to exudative AMD in the year 2001. This is expected to rise to approximately 500,000 per year by the year 2030.

Epidemiology and Etiology

Choroidal neovascularization is the leading cause of central blindness among the elderly in the United States and in most of the Western world. The pathophysiology of exudative AMD and the specific stimuli required for the development of CNV are not well understood.

Pathology

Choroidal neovascularization is typically derived from choroidal venules and may invade above and beneath the RPE through breaks in Bruch's membrane.

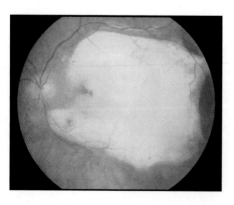

Figure 1-13   Disciform scar   *A large area of submacular fibrosis with chronic submacular fluid is noted. Disciform scarring is the final common pathway for exudative AMD. Visual acuity is counting fingers eccentrically.*

History

Patients with exudative AMD may note loss of vision, distortion of vision, or blurring of vision. Patients may be asymptomatic, however, if the fellow eye continues to function well. There may be a history of loss of vision in the fellow eye due to exudative AMD.

Clinical and Fluorescein Angiographic Signs

Classic Choroidal Neovascularization Fundus biomicroscopy may reveal a greenish-grey subretinal lesion often with associated submacular fluid, hemorrhage, or lipid exudation due to the incompetent vasculature of the CNV. Occasionally, a ring of dark pigment may surround the CNV. The pigment ring is more commonly observed in patients with classic CNV. Fluorescein angiography is necessary to characterize the nature and location of the CNV. Choroidal neovascularization may be subfoveal if localized beneath the geometric center of the fovea, juxtafoveal if localized from 1 to 199 μm from the foveal center, or extrafoveal if 200 μm or farther from the center of the fovea.

Classic CNV is characterized by early appearance of fluorescein leakage during the choroidal and retinal vascular filling phases of the fluorescein angiogram (Figure 1-14A–G). The leakage may be characterized by a lacy appearance of a network of blood vessels (but this is not requisite) and typically is fairly well delineated. More importantly, the lesion must demonstrate continued leakage through the recirculation and late phases of the fluorescein angiogram.

Occult Choroidal Neovascularization Fundus biomicroscopy may demonstrate irregular elevation of the RPE most commonly in association with submacular fluid, hemorrhage, or lipid exudation due to the incompetent vasculature of the CNV; less commonly, irregular elevation of the RPE alone may comprise the only clinical sign of occult CNV. Occult CNV is characterized by later appearing and less intense fluorescein angiographic leakage. One type of occult CNV, fibrovascular pigment epithelial detachment, is characterized by irregular stippled hyperfluorescence with mild leakage or staining of fluorescein dye in poorly demarcated boundaries of leakage (Figure 1-15A–C). The second type of occult CNV, late leakage of undetermined source, is characterized by leakage of fluorescein dye in the recirculation phase of the fluorescein angiogram associated with pooling of fluorescein dye in the subretinal space and areas of speckled hyperfluorescence (Figure 1-16A–D).

Most patients with exudative AMD demonstrate a combination of classic and occult CNV (Figure 1-17A–D). Characterization of the different types of CNV is important as management recommendations are based not only on the location of the lesion, but also on the nature of the CNV.

Fibrovascular Pigment Epithelial Detachment and Serous Pigment Epithelial Detachment Fibrovascular pigment epithelial detachment is a form of occult CNV. Purely serous pigment epithelial detachment is characterized by a blister-like elevation of sub-RPE fluid. Fundus biomicroscopy shows an orange ring that illuminates with a slit-lamp light beam. A serous pigment epithelial detachment is often associated with a serous detachment of the neurosensory macula as well. Fluorescein angiography shows a uniform rapid filling of fluorescein dye beneath the boundaries of the pigment epithelial detachment (Figure 1-18A–D). Fibrovascular pigment epithelial detachments may have associated serous retinal pigment epithelial detachments and are often denoted by a notch on the fluorescein angiogram (Figure 1-19A,B). The notch represents the CNV. Fibrovascular pigment epithelial detachments are more likely to have a serosanguineous component in the sub-RPE fluid, and this may be visualized ophthalmoscopically. Indocyanine green angiography may be helpful in imaging presumed CNV in the setting of occult CNV and pigment epithelial detachment (Figure 1-19C,D).

Retinal Pigment Epithelial Tears Retinal pigment epithelial tears may be observed in association with pigment epithelial detachments. A scrolled edge of RPE may be

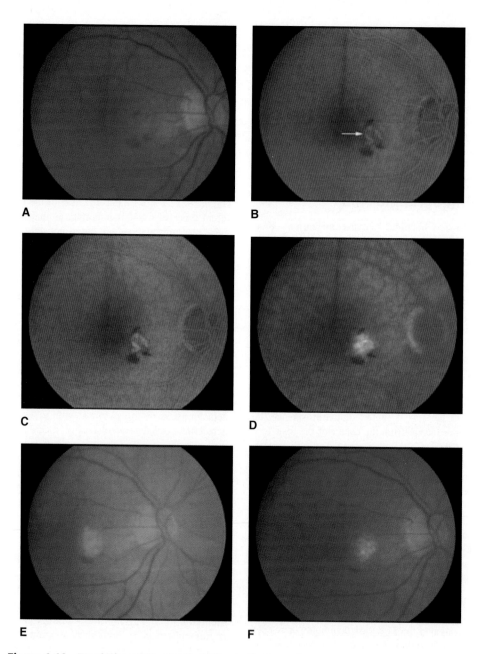

Figure 1-14   Exudative AMD, classic CNV   *A. Shallow submacular fluid and intraretinal hemorrhage is noted. B. Arterio-venous phase fluorescein angiogram showing a cartwheel of extrafoveal classic CNV (arrow) and hypofluorescence corresponding to retinal hemorrhage. C. Recirculation phase photograph showing early leakage of dye from the classic CNV. D. Late image showing some pooling of dye beneath the neurosensory retina. E. Thermal laser photocoagulation is performed and shows retinal whitening. F. Three weeks later there is evidence of atrophy in the area of laser treatment and resolution of the submacular fluid (continued).*

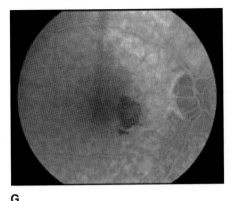

G

Figure 1-14 (cont.) *G. Fluorescein angiogram showing no evidence of recurrent CNV at 3 weeks. The patient remains at risk for the subsequent development of recurrent CNV.*

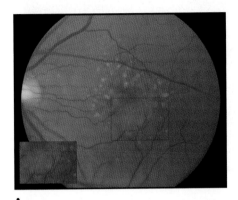

A

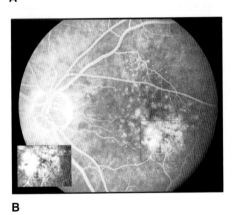

B

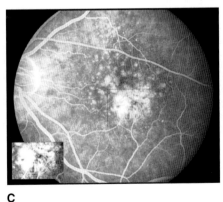

C

Figure 1-15   Occult CNV   *A. Color fundus photograph demonstrating drusen and slightly turbid submacular fluid centered inferior to the fovea (inset). **B.** Recirculation phase fluorescein angiogram demonstrating ill-defined stippled hyperfluorescence inferior to the fovea. There is some drusen staining as well (inset). **C.** Fluorescein angiogram demonstrating some mild leakage of fluorescein dye beneath the fovea. Late fluorescein angiographic images show ill-defined leakage inferior to the fovea (inset).*

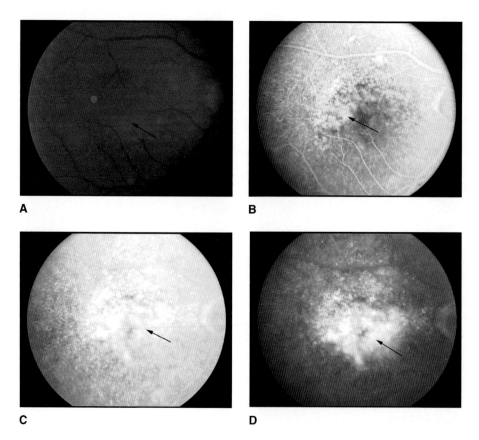

Figure 1-16 Occult CNV *A. Color fundus photograph showing turbid submacular fluid and drusen (arrow).* ***B.*** *Fluorescein angiogram showing ill-defined stippled hyperfluorescence temporal to the fovea (arrow).* ***C.*** *Fluorescein angiogram showing more diffuse ill-defined leakage (arrow).* ***D.*** *Late fluorescein angiogram showing poorly demarcated, stippled hyperfluorescence and leakage of dye characteristic of occult CNV (arrow).*

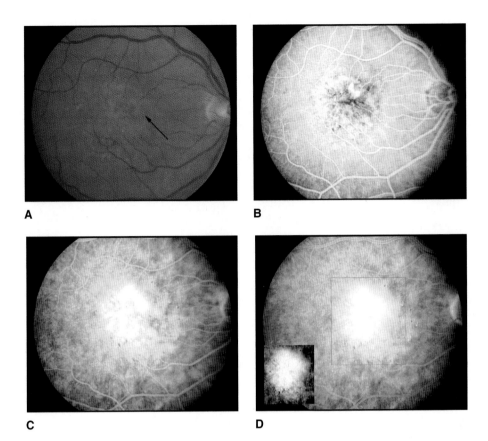

A   **B**

C   **D**

Figure 1-17   **Classic and occult CNV**   *A. Fundus photograph demonstrating macular edema as well as shallow submacular fluid due to exudative AMD* (arrow). *Some drusen are noted peripheral to the neurosensory detachment. **B.** Arterio-venous phase fluorescein angiogram showing hyperfluorescence consistent with combination of classic and occult CNV. Classic component is superior and temporal. **C.** Midphase fluorescein angiogram demonstrating leakage from the subfoveal CNV. Classic component shows brighter hyperfluorescence than the occult CNV. **D.** Pooling of fluorescein dye below the neurosensory detachment from classic and occult CNV* (inset).

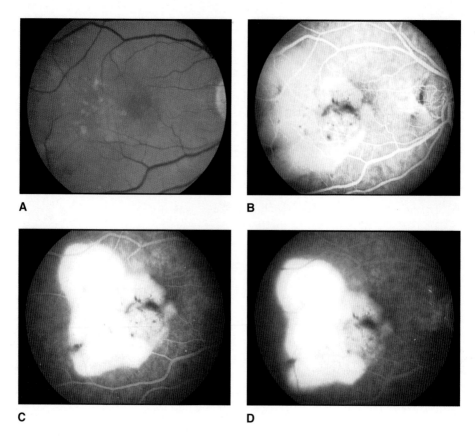

Figure 1-18   Retinal pigment epithelial detachment   *A. Color fundus photograph showing a retinal pigment epithelial detachment with submacular fluid centered temporal to the fovea. Some drusen are noted temporal to the detachment. **B.** Midphase fluorescein angiogram showing hyperfluorescence corresponding to a large retinal pigment epithelial detachment.*
*C. Recirculation phase fluorescein angiogram demonstrating pooling of dye beneath the pigment epithelial detachment and a fibrovascular component centered on the fovea. **D.** Fluorescein angiogram showing the extent of the serous and fibrovascular pigment epithelial detachment. The area of involvement remains unchanged from the recirculation phase image.*

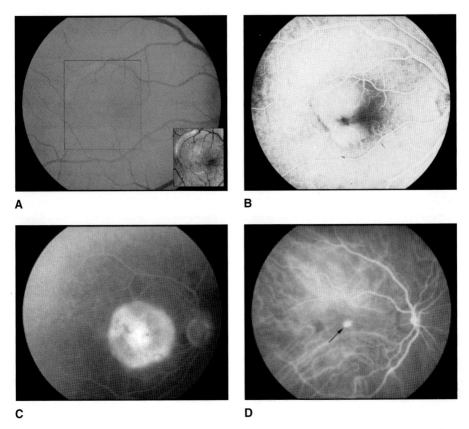

Figure 1-19 Serous pigment epithelial detachment *A. Color fundus photograph demonstrating a blister-like elevation of a serous pigment epithelial detachment* (inset). *B. Fluorescein angiogram showing a serous pigment epithelium detachment centered on the fovea with a notch on the nasal border. The notch may represent an area of CNV. C. Another patient with pigment epithelial detachment seen on fluorescein angiography; no notch is observed. D. Indocyanine green angiogram showing a focal area of hyperfluorescence* (arrow) *within the pigment epithelial detachment corresponding to presumed CNV.*

apparent with fundus biomicroscopy and sometimes is associated with a flattening of the retinal pigment epithelial detachment. Vision loss is typically observed with a retinal pigment epithelial tear, although in some cases, good central vision is preserved in the short term. Fluorescein angiography shows early intense hyperfluorescence corresponding to the area of denuded RPE and relative hypofluorescence where there is scrolled and redundant retinal pigment epithelial tissue (Figure 1-20A–D).

Submacular Hemorrhage A large submacular hemorrhage may be associated with apoplectic loss of central vision. It may be the presenting manifestation of exudative AMD or may follow the development of classic or occult CNV, or both (Figure 1-21). Fundus biomicroscopy shows subretinal and sometimes preretinal or subretinal pigment epithelial hemorrhage that may have significant elevation greater than 1 mm in height. The extent of the hemorrhage may be limited or sometimes can extend to involve the entire posterior pole

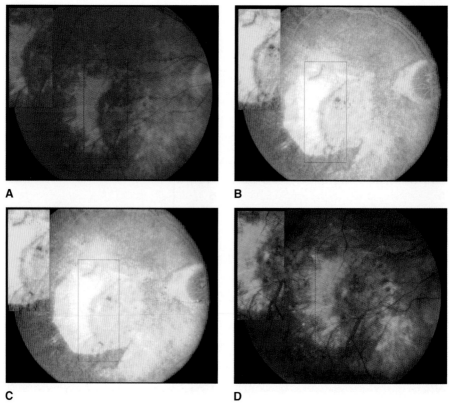

A **B**

C **D**

Figure 1-20 Retinal pigment epithelial tear *A. A retinal pigment epithelial tear is noted by the discrete borders of the loss of pigment in the temporal macula. A scrolled edge can be seen as a curved hyperpigmented line extending through the fovea (inset).* ***B.*** *Early-phase fluorescein angiogram showing a bright, well-delineated area of hyperfluorescence corresponding to the retinal pigment epithelial tear. The redundant scrolled edge of the tear shows as relative hypofluorescence in an arc through the fovea (inset).* ***C.*** *Late-phase fluorescein angiogram showing no evidence of fluorescein dye leakage beyond the temporal border of the tear (inset).* ***D.*** *Thirty months later, the color fundus photograph shows some submacular fibrosis and atrophy in the retinal pigment epithelial tear. Underlying choroidal vessels are visible in the region of the tear (inset).*

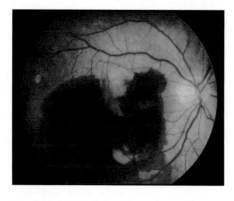

Figure 1-21 Submacular hemorrhage
Submacular hemorrhage can cause dramatic sudden loss of central vision in patients with exudative AMD. Note that some overlyings retinal vessels are visible, the clue that the hemorrhage is subretinal.

or beyond. Vision loss typically correlates with the extent of subfoveal involvement and the two-dimensional size of the submacular hemorrhage. The fluorescein angiography may or may not show source CNV. The submacular hemorrhage will typically obscure underlying normal and pathologic choroidal fluorescence.

Disciform Scar Disciform scar is the final common pathway of exudative AMD. Thin or thick fibrotic submacular scarring may be observed, and there may be associated chronic submacular fluid, lipid exudation, cystoid macular edema, and submacular hemorrhage (see Figure 1-13). Occasionally, retinochoroidal anastomoses are seen connecting the underlying pathologic CNV and fibrosis with the retinal circulation. Fluorescein angiography shows staining of the disciform scar and leakage from any residual active CNV.

Differential Diagnosis

Signs of exudative AMD such as retinal hemorrhage, lipid exudation, macular edema, and submacular fluid may be confused with non-AMD conditions. For example, serous detachments of the macula may be associated with central serous retinopathy, although this is typically seen in younger patients. Intraretinal hemorrhage can be seen in retinal venous occlusive disease, hypertensive retinopathy, or diabetic retinopathy, but it also may be the presenting sign of early CNV. Cystoid macular edema may be a presenting sign of CNV. Cystoid macular edema due to CNV may be confused with pseudophakic cystoid macular edema. Macular edema associated with retinal vascular conditions such as venous occlusive disease, parafoveal telangiectasia, or diabetic retinopathy may present in similar fashion to exudative AMD. Stereoscopic fluorescein angiography is critical to make the correct diagnosis. Polypoidal choroidal vasculopathy is an exudative maculopathy that may be seen in all races but usually is observed in African Americans or Asian Americans in whom exudative AMD is less common. This condition is characterized by choroidal aneurysms with associated serosanguineous pigment epithelial detachments and submacular exudation. This particular condition is imaged well with indocyanine green angiography, whereby choroidal saccular aneurysms may be highlighted in a peripapillary distribution or in a macular distribution. Large submacular or intraretinal hemorrhages can be seen in the setting of trauma, choroidal tumor, or retinal arterial macroaneurysm, and these conditions, in addition to exudative AMD, should be considered in the context of this clinical presentation.

Prognosis and Management

The visual prognosis of exudative AMD is poor with respect to central vision; peripheral vision typically remains unaffected. Seventy-five percent of eyes that develop exudative AMD will be legally blind (20/200 or worse) within 3 years. Classic CNV causes a more rapid visual decline than occult CNV; some eyes with occult CNV may retain reading vision for years. There are a variety of clinical research trials investigating new treatments for exudative AMD.

Evidence-based Therapies

THERMAL LASER PHOTOCOAGULATION The Macular Photocoagulation Study Group Classic has established that thermal laser photocoagulation is the treatment of choice for well-delineated extrafoveal CNV. The major problem with this therapy is that up to 60% of eyes will develop recurrent CNVs, the majority of which are subfoveal (Figure 1-22A,B). Well-defined juxtafoveal CNV may be treated by thermal laser photocoagulation or by photodynamic therapy (see next discussion).

VERTEPORFIN PHOTODYNAMIC THERAPY The Treatment of AMD with Photodynamic Therapy Study Group has established that verteporfin photodynamic therapy is the treatment of choice for predominantly classic subfoveal CNV. Although visual improvement is achieved in only a minority of eyes (approximately 15% at 1 year), treated eyes show more visual stability than observed eyes over 2 years. Treatment benefit has also been established for occult CNV but not for mixed lesions that are less than predominantly classic CNV (Figure 1-23A–F).

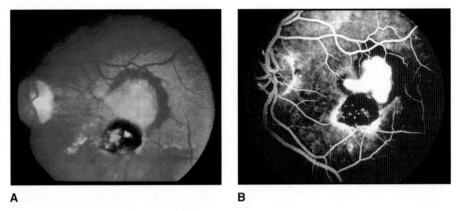

A

B

Figure 1-22   Recurrent CNV after thermal laser treatment   *A. Color fundus photograph shows prior area of hyperpigmented thermal laser photocoagulation scar and new submacular hemorrhage and fluid extending through the fovea. **B.** Fluorescein angiogram showing the hyperfluorescent, subfoveal, recurrent CNV surrounded by a rim of hypofluorescence. The old thermal laser scar is predominantly hypofluorescent inferior to the CNV.*

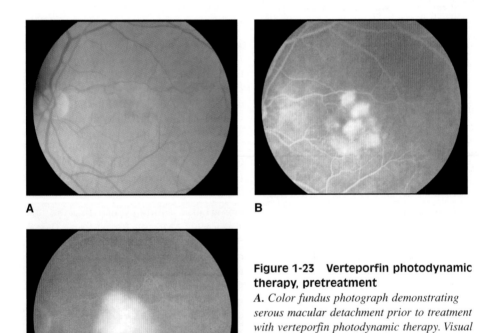

A

B

C

Figure 1-23   Verteporfin photodynamic therapy, pretreatment
*A. Color fundus photograph demonstrating serous macular detachment prior to treatment with verteporfin photodynamic therapy. Visual acuity was 20/80. **B.** Pretreatment fluorescein angiogram demonstrating predominantly classic subfoveal CNV. **C.** Pretreatment fluorescein angiogram demonstrating leakage within the neurosensory detachment.*

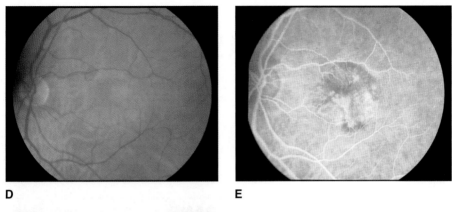

D

E

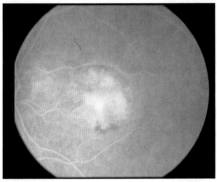

F

Figure 1-23   Verteporfin photodynamic therapy, posttreatment   D. *Posttreatment (3-month) color fundus photograph reveals diminished submacular fluid. Visual acuity was 20/50.* **E.** *Posttreatment fluorescein angiogram demonstrating less leakage.* **F.** *Posttreatment fluorescein angiogram demonstrating some staining of the CNV and minimal leakage of dye.*

Investigational Therapies The Submacular Surgery Trials are investigating surgical evacuation of large submacular hemorrhage and CNV. Retinal translocation surgery has shown the potential to improve central vision, but a surgical trial has not established this as a widespread technique. Pharmacologic interventions (angiostatic steroids, anticytokine drugs) are being explored alone and in combination with photodynamic therapy for subfoveal CNV. Displacement of large submacular hemorrhages with or without clot lysing agents such as tissue plasminogen activator may improve vision for some patients and may also reveal underlying CNV.

Chapter 2

MACULAR DISEASES

J. Arch McNamara, MD

MACULAR EPIRETINAL MEMBRANE

Definition

Macular epiretinal membrane is an acquired formation of a semitransparent fibrocellular membrane in the macula.

Epidemiology and Etiology

Macular epiretinal membranes may be either idiopathic or secondary to other intraocular abnormalities, including retinal breaks, retinal vascular disease, uveitis, blunt and penetrating trauma, and surgery. Idiopathic macular epiretinal membranes are most common after 50 years of age. Males and females are affected equally. Bilateral macular epiretinal membranes occur in approximately 20% of patients, with the severity of the membranes usually asymmetric. Most patients have posterior vitreous detachment (PVD), and it is thought that this phenomenon may contribute to formation of the membrane. After PVD, a portion of posterior cortical vitreous may be left behind on the macula, or the internal limiting membrane may be disrupted, allowing glial cells to proliferate on the surface of the retina. These proliferating glial cells form the epiretinal membrane. After retinal break formation and trauma, retinal pigment epithelial cells may escape into the vitreous cavity and settle upon the macula. These cells may then undergo metaplasia to glial cells, allowing the formation of macular epiretinal membranes.

History

If the macular epiretinal membrane is thin and not producing distortion of the retina, then the patient is usually asymptomatic. With progressive thickening and contraction of the membrane, patients begin to notice decreased vision, metamorphopsia, and macropsia or micropsia. Most patients maintain vision better than 6/15.

Important Clinical Signs

Macular epiretinal membranes initially appear as translucent, glistening membranes over, or adjacent to, the central macula (Figure 2-1). There may be a "pseudohole" appearance over the fovea. As the membrane matures, it becomes more opaque (Figure 2-2A). There may be associated superficial hemorrhages or nerve fiber layer infarcts. The membranes contract centrally and cause wrinkling and distortion of the underlying retina. This wrinkling and distortion gives rise to other names for this condition: cellophane maculopathy, surface

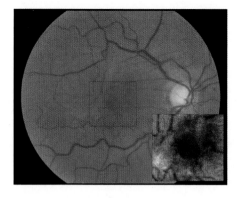

Figure 2-1   Macular epiretinal membrane   *Glistening membrane over the macula causing distortion of central retina* (inset).

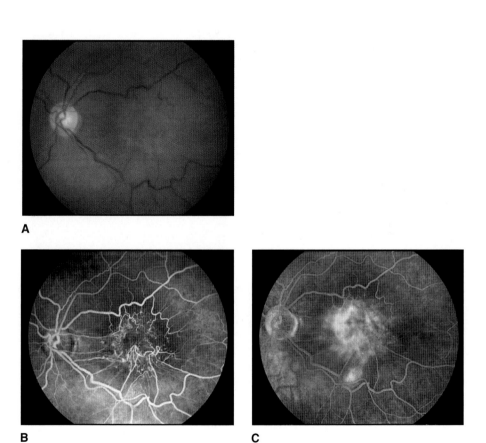

Figure 2-2   Macular epiretinal membrane   *A. Thick membrane over the macula causing distortion of the central retina. **B.** Fluorescein angiogram showing distortion of the macular retina. **C.** Late-phase fluorescein angiogram showing intraretinal leakage of dye from distorted retinal vessels.*

wrinkling retinopathy, and macular pucker. If the distortion is severe, cystoid macular edema and even shallow tractional retinal detachment can occur.

Differential Diagnosis

Cystoid macular edema
Choroidal neovascularization
Macular hole
Choroidal folds
Combined hamartoma of the retina
Retinal pigment epithelium

Diagnostic Evaluation

Usually measurement of visual acuity, Amsler grid testing (to assess for metamorphopsia, macropsia, or micropsia) and ophthalmoscopy suffice to make the diagnosis of macular epiretinal membrane. Slit-lamp biomicroscopy with either a noncontact or a contact lens greatly facilitates diagnosis. Fluorescein angiography will clearly delineate retinal vascular distortion and leakage that may occur from cystoid macular edema (Figure 2-2B,C).

Prognosis and Management

Most patients with uniocular macular epiretinal membrane and vision better that 6/15 are usually not significantly symptomatic and do not require intervention. Patients with vision of 6/18 or worse and those patients with intolerable distortion may benefit from pars plana vitrectomy with membrane peeling and removal (Figure 2-3A,B). Rarely the membrane may spontaneously release, leading to resolution of symptoms.

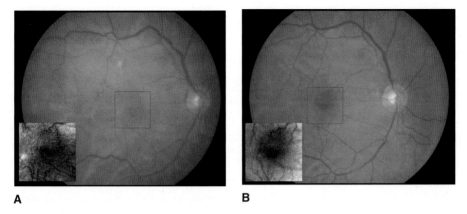

A   **B**

Figure 2-3   Macular epiretinal membrane   *A. Preoperative appearance of membrane* (inset); *visual acuity was 6/60. Note the retinal folds and retinal vascular compression and tortuosity. **B**. Postoperative appearance of membrane* (inset); *visual acuity was 6/12. There is less retinal vascular tortuosity.*

IDIOPATHIC MACULAR HOLE

Definition

Idiopathic macular hole is an acquired full-thickness defect of retina in the central macula.

Epidemiology and Etiology

Idiopathic macular holes typically occur in the sixth through eighth decades of life with a 3:1 predominance in women. The incidence of bilaterality is 5% to 10%. Tangential vitreoretinal traction is the presumed cause of development of idiopathic macular hole. The Gass classification of the stages of idiopathic macular hole development is helpful in understanding the progression of the disease and the biomicroscopic findings (Table 2-1).

Patients with a full-thickness macular hole in one eye and an impending macular hole with no PVD in the fellow eye are at substantial risk of progression to stage 2 macular hole in the second eye. Patients with a full-thickness macular hole in one eye and a normal retina with PVD in the fellow eye are at very little risk of progressing to macular hole in the second eye.

History

Patients usually report decreased visual acuity with central scotoma. There may be metamorphopsia. Often patients notice decreased vision in the affected eye when the fellow eye is incidentally covered as for a routine eye examination.

Important Clinical Signs

Depending on the stage and severity of the macular hole, the visual acuity may be near normal or severely reduced to less than 6/120. Amsler grid testing will often reveal metamorphopsia or a central scotoma. Ophthalmoscopy and slit-lamp biomicroscopy reveal findings consistent with the stage of the macular hole. Stage 1 holes appear as a small yellow cyst or ring around the fovea with a loss of the foveal depression (Figure 2-4). Stage 2 holes appear as a small round or crescent-shaped defect in the fovea (Figure 2-5). Stage 3 holes have a dark round defect in the fovea, often with a cuff of subretinal fluid accumulation (Figure 2-6). Stage 4 holes are often larger than stage 3 holes and are associated with a PVD (Figure 2-7). There are often small yellow dots in the center of the hole at the level of the retinal pigment epithelium (Figure 2-8).

TABLE 2-1   STAGES OF DEVELOPMENT OF IDIOPATHIC MACULAR HOLE

Stage 1A	Early contraction of outer part of vitreous cortex with foveolar detachment (impending macular hole)
Stage 1B	Further vitreous contraction and condensation of the prefoveal vitreous cortex with foveal detachment (impending macular hole)
Stage 2	Small (<400 μm) perifoveal dehiscence
Stage 3	Larger (>400 μm) central full-thickness hole usually accompanied by a rim of retinal elevation; the posterior cortical vitreous remains attached; there may be a small operculum overlying the macular hole
Stage 4	Macular hole has an associated complete posterior vitreous detachment; these holes are usually large (>400 μm).

Based on Gass JD. Reappraisal of biomicroscopic classification of stages of development of a macular hole. Am J Opthalmol 1995;119:752–759.

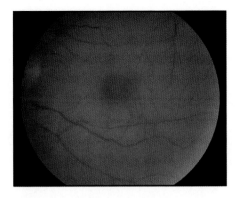

Figure 2-4   Idiopathic macular hole, stage 1B   *Stage 1B macular hole with yellow ring appearance around the fovea. Visual acuity remains 6/7.5.*

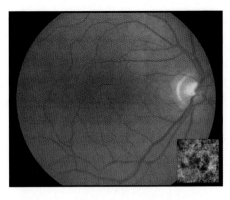

Figure 2-5   Idiopathic macular hole, stage 2   *Stage 2 macular hole appears as a small round defect in the fovea* (inset).

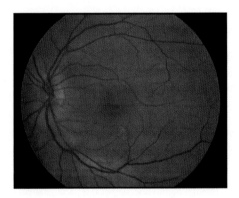

Figure 2-6   Idiopathic macular hole, stage 3   *Stage 3 macular hole with cuff of subretinal fluid around the hole.*

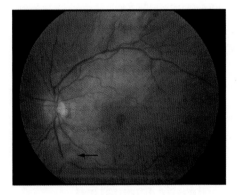

Figure 2-7   Idiopathic macular hole, stage 4   *Stage 4 macular hole; note condensed vitreous of posterior vitreous detachment overlying inferotemporal vascular arcade* (arrow).

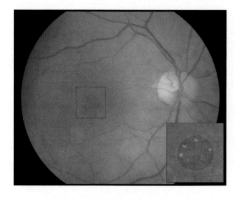

Figure 2-8   Idiopathic macular hole, stage 4
Stage 4 macular hole with subretinal precipitates (inset).

Associated Clinical Signs

The Watzke-Allen sign is the patient's description of discontinuance in the center of a thin slit beam shone over the fovea.

Differential Diagnosis

Macular epiretinal membrane with pseudo-hole
Cystoid macular edema
Central serous retinopathy
Choroidal neovascular membrane
Solar retinopathy

Diagnostic Evaluation

Clinical examination alone is often diagnostic. Fluorescein angiography in eyes with stage 2, 3, or 4 macular holes will reveal early central hyperfluorescence in the fovea corresponding to loss of xanthophyll pigment and retinal pigment epithelial depigmentation and atrophy at the base of the hole. Optical coherence tomography may be used in equivocal cases (Figure 2-9).

Prognosis and Management

No treatment is recommended for stage 1 macular holes because these resolve spontaneously 50% of the time. Spontaneous resolution of more advanced stages of macular hole can occur, but it is rare. Vitrectomy for more advanced stages of macular hole can be performed. The surgery consists of a standard pars plana vitrectomy, peeling of the posterior hyaloid, and injection of a long-acting gas such as perfluoropropane. Peeling of the internal membrane may also be done. Patients must then maintain face-down positioning for 1 to 2 weeks to allow the gas bubble to tamponade the hole. The hole can be closed and vision improved with a success rate of 80% to 90% (Figure 2-10A,B).

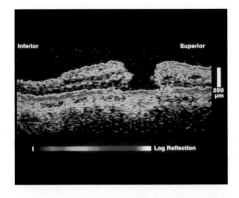

Figure 2-9   Idiopathic macular hole, OCT image   *Optical coherence tomography (OCT) of stage 4 macular hole showing complete defect in retina. (Courtesy of the New England Eye Center.)*

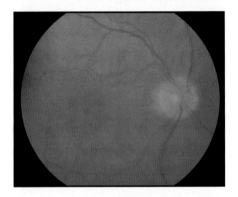

Figure 2-10A   Idiopathic macular hole, preoperative   *Preoperative appearance of stage 3 macular hole (yellow spots are incidental drusen).*

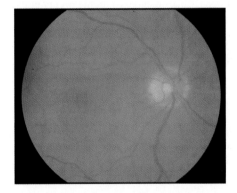

Figure 2-10B   Idiopathic macular hole, postoperative   *Postoperative appearance of stage 3 macular hole; note closed appearance of hole. Vision improved to 6/12 from 6/30.*

VITREOMACULAR TRACTION SYNDROME

Definition

Vitreomacular traction syndrome is an acquired condition in which there is partial separation of the posterior hyaloid with persistent attachment to the macula and, occasionally, the optic nerve head.

Epidemiology and Etiology

Vitreomacular traction syndrome occurs in the same age group as those who develop PVD. Posterior vitreous detachment is uncommon before 50 years of age and is present in over 50% of people aged 70 years and older.

History

Patients who have vitreomacular traction syndrome experience progressive distortion and visual loss, which is often more severe than that occurring with macular epiretinal membrane.

Important Clinical Signs

The posterior hyaloid is visibly thickened. There is macular distortion, often with tractional retinal detachment in the macula. Retinal striae may be present. There may be traction in the peripapillary region. An epiretinal membrane may be seen clinically (Figure 2-11).

Differential Diagnosis

Macular epiretinal membrane
Combined hamartoma of the retina and retinal pigment epithelium

Diagnostic Evaluation

Fluorescein angiography may reveal retinal vascular distortion and leakage. There may be cystoid macular edema and optic nerve edema. Ultrasonography and optical coherence tomography may help determine the presence of tractional retinal detachment.

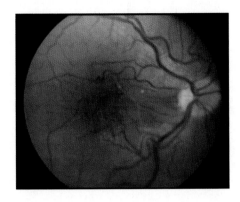

Figure 2-11   Vitreomacular traction syndrome   *Adhesion of the vitreous to a premacular membrane elevates the fovea and creates macular distortion.*

Prognosis and Management

Rarely patients may experience spontaneous improvement if posterior vitreous detachment occurs. Surgical intervention is indicated if visual acuity is reduced to 6/21 or worse. During vitrectomy surgery, the posterior hyaloid is removed, as are any epiretinal membranes in the macular region. The retinal architecture can be restored to a normal appearance. The vision can be improved but usually complete recovery does not occur due to residual macular edema.

CYSTOID MACULAR EDEMA

Definition

Cystoid macular edema (CME) is the result of accumulation of intraretinal fluid in the perifoveal region. Fluid accumulates in cystic spaces that may be visible clinically and on fluorescein angiography.

Epidemiology and Etiology

Cystoid macular edema is most commonly seen after cataract surgery. Other types of ocular surgery, such as trabeculectomy, laser photocoagulation and cryoretinopexy, may also give rise to CME. Less commonly, CME is seen in association with diabetic retinopathy, choroidal neovascularization, uveitis, retinal vein obstruction, perifoveal telangiectasis, retinitis pigmentosa, and other entities.

History

Cystoid macular edema following cataract surgery typically has its onset 6 to 10 weeks after surgery. Patients experience an initial improvement in vision only to be followed by decreasing central vision in the range of 6/12 to 6/30.

Important Clinical Signs

When CME is present in the post–cataract surgery patient, there is often no abnormality noted in the anterior segment. On slit-lamp biomicroscopy, patients will have cystic spaces in the perifoveal area (Figure 2-12A), best seen by narrowing the slit beam adjacent to the fovea. There will also be thickening of the central macula and, occasionally, tiny round intraretinal hemorrhages at the edge of the foveal avascular zone.

Associated Clinical Signs

There may be no associated clinical signs when CME occurs after cataract surgery. However, CME is more common after complicated cataract surgery in which there has been rupture of the posterior capsule and vitreous loss. Such findings as vitreous to the wound, iris to the wound, iris atrophy, and an opening in the posterior capsule may therefore be present.

When CME is present in association with other ophthalmic diseases, then the findings of those entities will be present. For example, pigment migration into the retinal midperiphery will be present in patients with CME in association with retinitis pigmentosa, and diffuse intraretinal hemorrhages will be present in patients with CME in association with retinal venous occlusive disease.

Differential Diagnosis

Choroidal neovascularization
Diabetic macular edema

Diagnostic Evaluation

Fluorescein angiography is helpful in establishing the diagnosis of CME. Fluorescein angiography shows accumulation of dye in the perifoveal region in a petalloid pattern (Figure 2-12B). There is often leakage of dye from the optic nerve head (Figure 2-12C). The foveal avascular zone is not enlarged in uncomplicated CME.

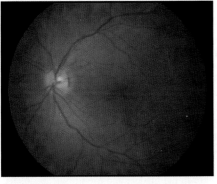

A

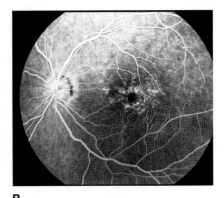

B

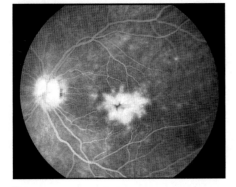

C

Figure 2-12   Cystoid macular edema
*A. The normal foveal reflex is lost and there are cystoid changes in the central macula. **B.** Early arteriovenous transit phase fluorescein angiogram showing leakage of dye in the perifoveal area. **C.** Late-phase fluorescein angiogram showing "petalloid" pattern of dye leakage in addition to leakage of dye from the optic nerve head.*

Angiographic CME may be present in as many as 60% of patients following cataract surgery. Clinically significant CME, in which patients are symptomatic, occurs in 2% to 10% of patients following uncomplicated cataract surgery.

Prognosis and Management

Most patients who suffer postoperative CME will undergo spontaneous resolution within 6 months. Therapeutic intervention is indicated if patients are symptomatic with decreased vision.

There is no single accepted regimen for management of postoperative CME. The most common therapies are topical or periocular corticosteroids, topical nonsteroidal anti-inflammatory drugs, and oral carbonic anhydrase inhibitors in various frequencies of administration and combination of agents.

Surgical intervention with Nd:YAG laser vitreolysis for thin strands of vitreous trapped in the cataract wound or vitrectomy for more extensive vitreous or iris incarceration or vitreomacular adhesion may result in resolution of CME.

POLYPOIDAL CHOROIDAL VASCULOPATHY

Definition

Polypoidal choroidal vasculopathy (PCV) is an idiopathic hemorrhagic disorder of the macula.

Epidemiology and Etiology

Polypoidal choroidal vasculopathy is a disorder of the inner choroidal vasculature in which there is a network of branching vessels deep to the choriocapillaris in association with terminal aneurysmal dilations. It is assumed that PCV represents a form of choroidal neovascularization (CNV). However, polypoidal CNV behaves differently from other forms of CNV, and the visual prognosis is better compared with CNV.

Polypoidal choroidal vasculopathy was initially described in elderly black women but is now known to occur in all races with preponderance in heavily pigmented individuals. Men are equally affected as women. The average age of onset of polypoidal CNV is much younger than that of age-related macular degeneration, but the range of age at onset is wider (less than 25 to more than 85 years). Lesions are usually bilateral, but patients have been followed for years with unilateral involvement.

History

Patients with PCV present with decreased and distorted vision if serosanguineous complications occur in the macula.

Important Clinical Signs

Patients with PCV may develop chronic recurrent acute serosanguineous detachments of the retina and retinal pigment epithelium. The vascular lesions may be seen with slit-lamp biomicroscopy as reddish orange spheroidal or polypoidal lesions. The lesions have a predilection for the peripapillary area but may be seen elsewhere in the macula and even in the periphery. Rarely, bullous or total serosanguineous retinal detachment with or without vitreous hemorrhage may occur.

Associated Clinical Signs

Systemic hypertension is often associated with severe PCV with visual loss.

Differential Diagnosis

Age-related macular degeneration with choroidal neovascularization
Central serous choroidopathy
Retinal pigment epithelial detachment

Diagnostic Evaluation

Serosanguineous detachments of the retina and retinal pigment epithelium may be seen clinically (Figure 2-13A). Fluorescein angiography is usually not an effective imaging

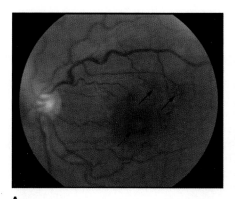

A

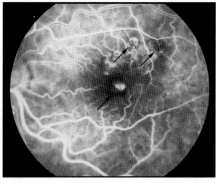

B

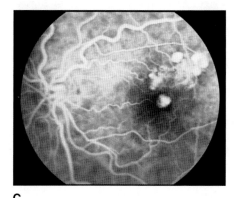

C

Figure 2-13   Polypoidal choroidal vasculopathy (PCV) *A. Areas of serosanguineous retinal detachment in the macula* (arrows). *B. Venous filling phase fluorescein angiogram showing network of branching choroidal vessels* (arrows). *C. Late-phase fluorescein angiogram showing leakage of dye in the choroid and terminal aneurysmal dilations.*

technique, because the fluorescence of the choriocapillaris often masks the vascular lesions (Figure 2-13B,C). Indocyanine green angiography, which better images the choroid, often provides the best visualization of the active lesions.

Prognosis and Management

The serosanguineous lesions may resolve spontaneously without progressing to fibrous proliferation. The vascular lesions may involute during periods of disease inactivity, making diagnosis difficult. In contrast, the vascular lesions may continue to grow and repeatedly bleed. These lesions may then develop fibrovascular scarring. Patients may suffer severe visual loss. Treatment for systemic hypertension, if associated with PCV, may be important in limiting the severity of the disease.

Laser photocoagulation can be considered, especially for serosanguineous complications under the fovea. Treatment to the active polypoidal CNV or to the aneurysmal changes outside the fovea often leads to regression of the entire lesion. This is unlike the experience with CNV due to age-related macular degeneration, in which the entire lesion must be treated to prevent further hemorrhagic complications. Ocular photodynamic therapy may be considered for subfoveal lesions.

DEGENERATIVE MYOPIA

Definition

Degenerative myopia describes a retinal degenerative condition that consists of thinning of the retinal pigment epithelium and choroid, retinal pigment epithelial atrophy, CNV, and subretinal hemorrhage in patients with progressive elongation of the eye from myopia usually greater than −6 diopters.

Epidemiology and Etiology

The prevalence of degenerative myopia varies among different races and ethnic groups. Degenerative myopia is more prevalent in women than in men.

History

Patients with degenerative myopia may slowly lose central vision due to progressive atrophy of the macular region. More abrupt vision loss may occur from macular subretinal hemorrhage or CNV. Spontaneous improvement in vision may occur if subretinal hemorrhage not associated with CNV resorbs.

Important Clinical Signs

The clinical findings of degenerative myopia are thought to be due to progressive elongation of the globe. The hallmark finding is the so-called myopic crescent of retinal pigment epithelial atrophy adjacent to the optic nerve (Figure 2-14A). This atrophic area is usually at the temporal aspect of the disc. However, the atrophy may be located anywhere around the circumference of the disc and may extend through the central macula. The disc itself may be vertically elongated or tilted, or both (Figure 2-14B).

Central macular abnormalities may lead to visual loss. Gyrate areas of atrophy in the posterior pole may involve the foveal region. Lacquer cracks, which are spontaneous linear breaks in Bruch's membrane, may be located in the fovea (see Figure 2-14B). Lacquer cracks are present in 4% of highly myopic eyes. Spontaneous subretinal hemorrhage without CNV may arise from lacquer cracks (Figure 2-14C). Fuchs' spots are round areas of subretinal hyperpigmentation, occasionally with surrounding atrophy, that are thought to

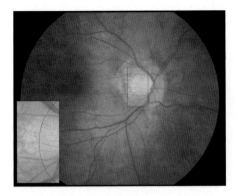

Figure 2-14A   Degenerative myopia, myopic crescent   *Temporal myopic crescent. Note "thinning" of retinal pigment epithelium (*inset *reveals true borders of optic nerve).*

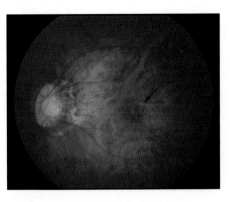

Figure 2-14B   Degenerative myopia, tilted disc   *Prominent tilted disc with temporal crescent and lacquer crack above fovea* (arrow).

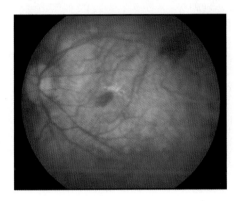

Figure 2-14C   Degenerative myopia, retinal hemorrhage   *Spontaneous subretinal (foveal) hemorrhage from lacquer crack without choroidal neovascularization (CNV).*

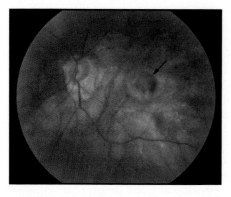

Figure 2-14D Degenerative myopia, CNV
Subfoveal CNV (arrow) *with pigmentation and shallow subretinal fluid.*

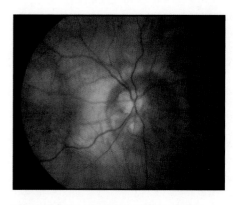

Figure 2-14E Degenerative myopia, posterior staphyloma *A staphyloma is present around the optic nerve.*

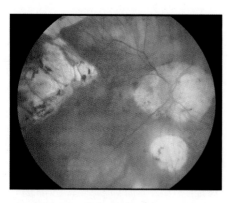

Figure 2-14F Degenerative myopia
Extensive chorioretinal atrophy in posterior pole and periphery in right eye.

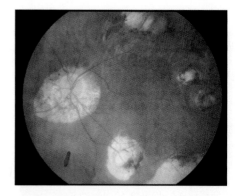

Figure 2-14G Degenerative myopia
Extensive chorioretinal atrophy in posterior pole and periphery in left eye.

represent areas of previous subretinal hemorrhage or CNV. Fuchs' spots are seen in 10% of highly myopic eyes after the age of 30.

Associated Clinical Signs

Choroidal neovascularization develops in 5% to 10% of eyes with an axial length greater than 26.5 mm (Figure 2-14D). Choroidal neovascularization is often seen in association with lacquer cracks. Posterior pole staphyloma, an excavation in the posterior pole associated with chorioretinal atrophy, may be present (Figure 2-14E).

Diffuse pigmentary alteration and patchy or diffuse areas of chorioretinal degeneration may be present in the retinal periphery (Figure 2-14F,G). Posterior vitreous detachment is more common and occurs at an earlier age in patients with degenerative myopia. Although lattice degeneration is not more common in degenerative myopia, patients are at an increased risk of retinal tear and retinal detachment.

Differential Diagnosis

Tilted disc syndrome
Optic disc coloboma
Presumed ocular histoplasmosis
Age-related macular degeneration
Gyrate atrophy

Diagnostic Evaluation

History, refractive error, and axial length measurement in association with the myriad findings on ophthalmoscopy all aid in the diagnosis of degenerative myopia. Fluorescein angiography is helpful to assess for CNV.

Prognosis and Management

There are no proven therapies to prevent the progression of myopia and its degenerative effects upon the retina. Scleral reinforcement and resection techniques have been reported to limit the elongation of the globe, but stabilization or improvement in vision has not been decisively demonstrated.

Laser photocoagulation should be considered carefully in patients with CNV in association with myopia. The CNV often remains small without treatment, and spreading of the atrophic photocoagulation lesion may lead to further visual loss. Ocular photodynamic therapy with verteporfin for subfoveal CNV may be useful. CNV lesions in degenerative myopia, in distinction from those in age-related macular degeneration, may remain stable without significant visual loss when no treatment is applied.

ANGIOID STREAKS

Definition

Angioid streaks are red or brown irregular lines that radiate from the optic nerve head. They represent breaks in thickened and calcified Bruch's membrane.

Epidemiology and Etiology

Angioid streaks are idiopathic 50% of the time but are also seen in association with certain systemic diseases (Table 2-2). The systemic disease most commonly associated with angioid streaks is pseudoxanthoma elasticum, or Grönblad-Strandberg syndrome. Other systemic conditions associated with angioid streaks are Paget's disease of bone, sickle cell anemia, and Ehlers-Danlos syndrome.

History

Patients are asymptomatic unless they develop CNV in association with their angioid streaks. When CNV develops, patients complain of decreased and distorted central vision.

Important Clinical Signs

Angioid streaks may appear as light red-orange to dark red-brown. The streaks may form a concentric ring around the optic nerve (Figure 2-15). They may extend through the macula and into the periphery. They may be thin or four times the width of retinal vessels. They are usually bilateral. Over time the streaks may become more atrophic.

Associated Clinical Signs

Choroidal neovascularization can be associated with angioid streaks (Figure 2-16A,B) and is the leading cause of vision loss due to rupture of the CNV, subretinal hemorrhage, and scarring (Figure 2-17).

Patients with pseudoxanthoma elasticum may have an additional fundus finding. There may be a fine stippled appearance to the fundus referred to as *peau d'orange* (like skin of an orange) most commonly seen in the temporal midperiphery (Figure 2-18A,B). Patients with this disease have abnormal dermal elastic tissue. They have loose skin folds in the neck and on the flexor aspects of joints. They may suffer cardiovascular disease from abnormal elastic tissue in blood vessel walls. They may develop gastrointestinal bleeding.

Patients with Paget's disease (osteitis deformans) have abnormal bone destruction and formation. They typically suffer from headache, enlarged skull, enlarged digits, bone fractures, and cardiovascular complications. Approximately 10% of patients with Paget's disease develop angioid streaks late in the course of their disease. These patients may also suffer visual loss from optic nerve compression by enlarging bone.

Angioid streaks develop in 1% to 2% of patients with sickle cell hemoglobinopathy. Patients with Ehlers-Danlos syndrome have hyperelasticity of the skin and hyperflexibility of the joints due to abnormal collagen organization.

TABLE 2-2 **SYSTEMIC ASSOCIATIONS WITH ANGIOID STREAKS**

Pseudoxanthoma elasticum (Grönblad-Strandberg syndrome)
Paget's disease (osteitis deformans)
Sickle cell hemoglobinopathy
Ehlers-Danlos syndrome

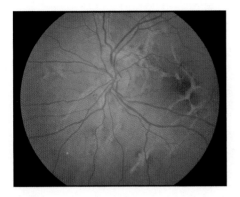

Figure 2-15 Angioid streaks, orange streaks *Orange lines around the optic nerve with extensions throughout the posterior pole.*

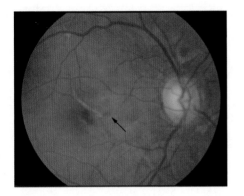

Figure 2-16A Angioid streaks, subretinal hemorrhage *Subretinal hemorrhage and retinal elevation adjacent to angioid streak is highly suggestive of CNV (arrow).*

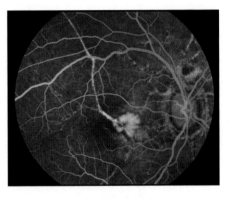

Figure 2-16B Angioid streaks, CNV *Fluorescein angiogram confirms CNV.*

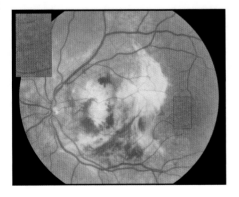

Figure 2-17 Angioid streaks, macular scarring *Severe macular scarring after rupture of CNV and hemorrhage (note* peau d'orange *appearance temporally; inset).*

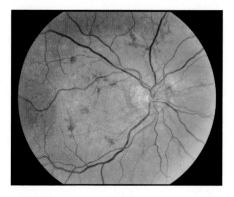

Figure 2-18A   Angioid streaks, subretinal hemorrhage *Pigmented streaks with sub-retinal hemorrhage.*

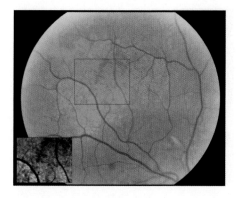

Figure 2-18B   Angioid streaks, peau d'orange Peau d'orange *appearance* (inset) *in superotemporal periphery.*

Differential Diagnosis

Traumatic choroidal rupture

Diagnostic Evaluation

In the early phase of fluorescein angiography angioid streaks appear as hyperfluorescent lines due to atrophy of the overlying retinal pigment epithelium. As in any condition associated with disruption of Bruch's membrane, CNV may occur. Typical findings of early hyperfluorescence of CNV with leakage may be seen on fluorescein angiography.

Prognosis and Management

When patients have angioid streaks, they remain at risk for CNV. There are no measures available to prevent the development of CNV. If patients develop extrafoveal or juxtafoveal CNV, standard laser photocoagulation can be considered. Ocular photodynamic therapy may become useful for patients with subfoveal CNV in association with angioid streaks.

Patients with angioid streaks should be particularly cautious regarding ocular trauma (Figure 2-19A–C). Safety glasses should be worn because these patients are more susceptible to choroidal rupture and hemorrhage from direct blows to the eye. Patients with angioid streaks should have a general medical evaluation to assess for systemic associations, especially because some of the manifestations, such as cardiovascular disease and gastrointestinal bleeding, are potentially life threatening.

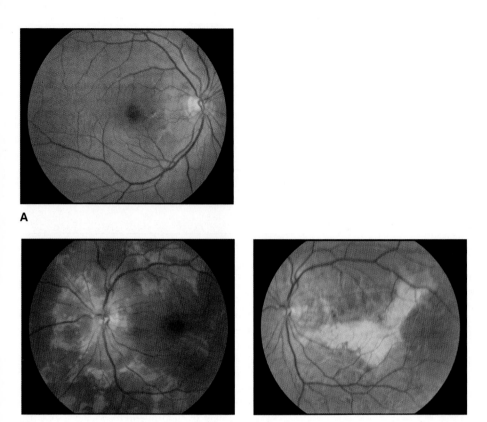

Figure 2-19   Angioid streaks, traumatic subretinal hemorrhage   *Patient with bilateral angioid streaks (**A**, right eye; **B**, left eye) was punched in the left eye and suffered extensive subretinal hemorrhage. The subretinal hemorrhage eventually resolved, but left severe scarring (**C**) and visual loss.*

CENTRAL SEROUS RETINOPATHY

Definition

Central serous retinopathy (CSR) is a disease in which a circumscribed serous detachment of the neurosensory retina develops, usually confined to the posterior pole. There may be an associated serous detachment of the retinal pigment epithelium. Central serous retinopathy is usually an idiopathic condition but may be seen in the setting of corticosteroid use.

Epidemiology and Etiology

Central serous retinopathy usually occurs in healthy middle-aged men, although women may also be affected. The exact etiology of CSR is unknown. A diffuse abnormality of the retinal pigment epithelium and choroid is likely because fluid resorption is impaired.

Central serous retinopathy is reportedly more common in patients with a so-called type A personality. Patients being treated with corticosteroids can have particularly severe CSR.

History

Patients may be asymptomatic unless the central macula is involved. Symptomatic patients experience sudden onset of decreased central vision with metamorphopsia. There may be macropsia or micropsia. Color vision is often affected, and patients may notice a relative scotoma.

Important Clinical Signs

On fundus examination patients will have an elevation in the macula due to serous detachment (Figure 2-20).

Associated Clinical Signs

There may be yellow spots; subretinal precipitates of fibrin deep to the detached retina (Figure 2-21). Often patients will have pigment epithelial clumping from prior episodes in either the involved or the fellow eye, or both (Figure 2-22). Occasionally patients will have an associated serous detachment of the retinal pigment epithelium (Figure 2-23A,B).

Rarely patients will have diffuse detachment of the posterior pole with gravity-dependent pooling of fluid inferiorly (Figure 2-24A–D). This may lead to "gutters" of retinal pigment epithelial alterations created by subretinal fluid that gravitates inferiorly.

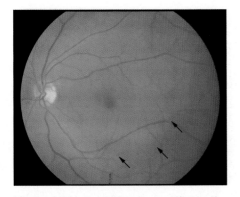

Figure 2-20　Central serous retinopathy (CSR), serous macular detachment
*Serous detachment in the macula (*arrow *denotes inferior and temporal border of the neurosensory detachment).*

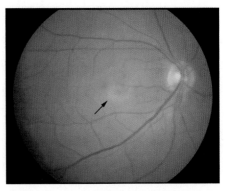

Figure 2-21　CSR, fibrin formation
*Subretinal fibrin precipitation in serous detachment of the macula (*arrow*).*

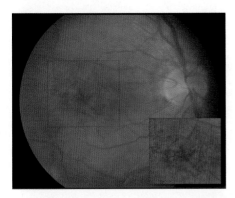

Figure 2-22　CSR, retinal pigment epithelial alterations　*Retinal pigment epithelial clumping in the macula following resolution of serous detachment (*inset*).*

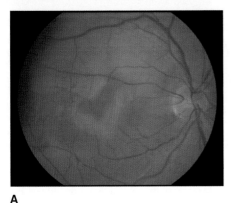

A

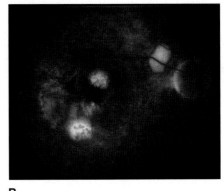

B

Figure 2-23　CSR　*A. Earlier phase of disease in same patient as in* **Figure 2-22**. *Note serous detachment of the retinal pigment epithelial superotemporal to the optic nerve and fibrin accumulation in the serous detachment of the macula.* **B.** *Fluorescein angiogram confirms serous detachment of retinal pigment epithelium adjacent to optic nerve.*

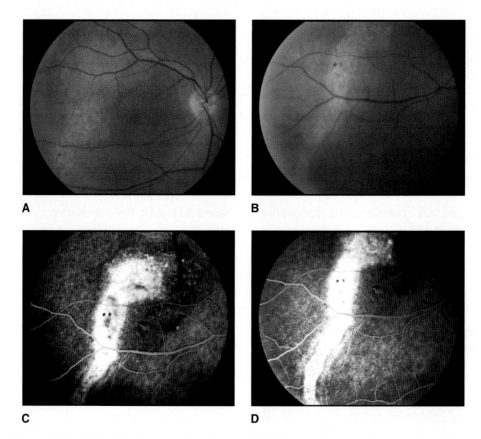

Figure 2-24 CSR *A,B.* *Patient with recurrent CSR (note small serous detachment of macula) who had prior episode(s) of serous detachment that led to gravity-dependent pooling of fluid inferiorly as evidenced by retinal pigment epithelial alterations extending into the inferior periphery.* *C,D.* *Fluorescein angiogram showing hyperfluorescence extending from the macula to the inferior periphery due to retinal pigment epithelial alterations from fluid pooling.*

Differential Diagnosis

Choroidal neovascularization, especially in older patients

Optic nerve pit with neurosensory macular retinal detachment

Posterior scleritis

Harada's disease

Rhegmatogenous retinal detachment

Circumscribed choroidal hemangioma

Amelanotic choroidal melanoma

Diagnostic Evaluation

A variety of fluorescein angiographic alterations may be seen in CSR. An expanding dot of hyperfluorescence is the most common alteration (Figure 2-25A–D). As the angiogram progresses, there is a spot of increasing hyperfluorescence at the level of the retinal pigment epithelium. In the late phase of the study, there is pooling of dye in the neurosensory detachment. Another less common pattern of hyperfluorescence is a

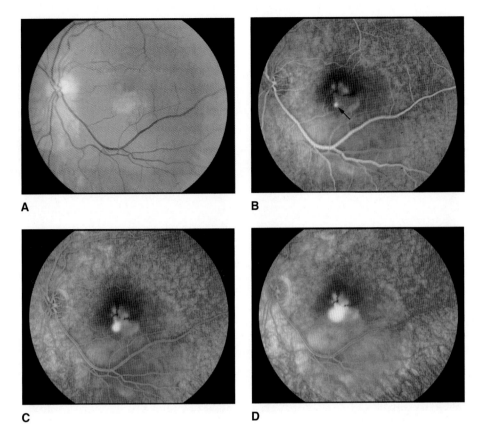

Figure 2-25   CSR   *A. Large serous detachment of the macula with fibrin under retina.*
B–D. Progressive enlargement of spot of hyperfluorescence on fluorescein angiography (arrow).

"smokestack" appearance in which dye spreads vertically from the retinal pigment epithelium (Figure 2-26A–D). Occasionally, multiple leakage spots will be seen.

Prognosis and Management

Most patients undergo spontaneous resolution in 1 to 3 months. However, there may be mild residual symptoms, including decreased central acuity, reduced contrast sensitivity, decreased color vision, and metamorphopsia. Rarely, patients have severe visual loss. Recurrences happen in 20% to 40% of patients.

If patients have persistent decreased vision with persistent fluid beyond 3 to 4 months, photocoagulation can be offered to the leak spot seen on fluorescein angiography (Figure 2-27). Patients with occupational needs for improved vision or return of stereoacuity can be considered for earlier treatment. Careful follow-up after laser photocoagulation is necessary because patients may develop CNV at the treatment site.

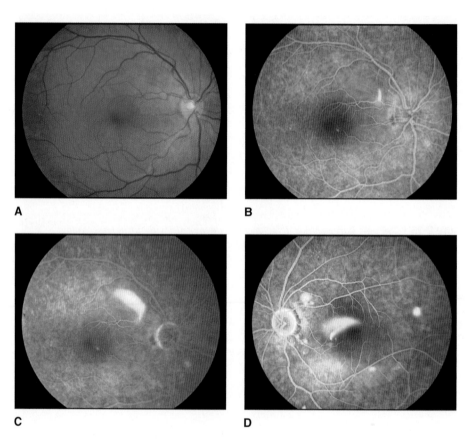

Figure 2-26   CSR, "smokestack" leakage   *A. Small serous detachment of the macula with retinal pigment epithelial alterations. **B,C.** "Smokestack" appearance of dye leakage on fluorescein angiography. **D.** Fluorescein angiogram showing multiple leakage spots of both the expanding dot and "smokestack" type of leakage.*

CHAPTER 2.   MACULAR DISEASES

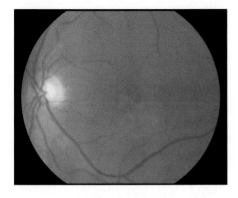

Figure 2-27   CSR, post–laser treatment
*Same patient as in **Figure 2-26** 10 weeks after laser photocoagulation. Note complete resolution of subretinal fluid but residual retinal pigment epithelial alterations. Vision improved from 6/30 to 6/9.*

CHOROIDAL FOLDS

Definition

Folding or wrinkling of the inner choroid, Bruch's membrane, retinal pigment epithelium, and inner retina is known as choroidal or chorioretinal folds.

Epidemiology and Etiology

Choroidal folds are usually idiopathic, but they can be seen in association with other ocular abnormalities (Table 2-3). They may be unilateral or bilateral.

History

Patients with long-standing choroidal folds are usually entirely asymptomatic. Those with acute onset of folds are usually symptomatic, with decreased vision and metamorphopsia.

Important Clinical Signs

Alternating light and dark streaks are seen in the posterior pole in patients with choroidal folds (Figure 2-28A). The folds may be horizontal, vertical, or oblique in orientation (Figure 2-28B).

Associated Clinical Signs

There may be no associated findings if the folds are idiopathic or associated with hyperopia. If there is another ocular condition, then there may be additional signs related to the cause of the folds, such as proptosis in association with an orbital tumor.

Differential Diagnosis

Retinal folds (e.g., from macular epiretinal membrane or retinal detachment)

Diagnostic Evaluation

On fluorescein angiography, alternating hyperfluorescent and hypofluorescent bands are seen. The crests of the folds are hyperfluorescent, and the troughs hypofluorescent (Figure 2-28C).

Prognosis and Management

There is no specific treatment for choroidal folds. If the folds are associated with another ocular condition, such as an orbital tumor or posterior scleritis, then the underlying cause of the choroidal folds should be treated.

TABLE 2-3   CAUSES OF CHOROIDAL FOLDS

Idiopathic
Hyperopia
Orbital tumors
Posterior scleritis
Scleral buckling surgery
Choroidal tumors
Hypotony
Choroidal neovascularization
Chorioretinal scarring

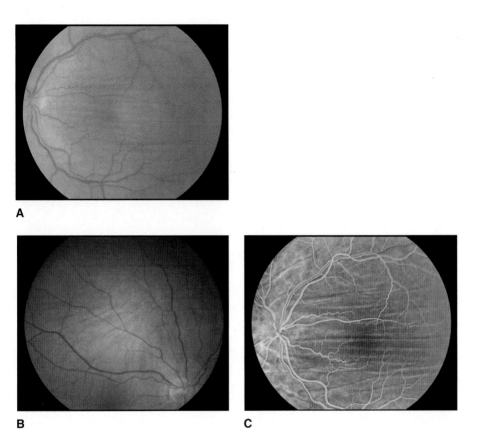

Figure 2-28 Choroidal folds *A. Alternating light and dark streaks through the macula. B. Obliquely oriented alternating light and dark streaks above the macula. C. Fluorescein angiogram of same patient as in (A). Note alternating hyperfluorescent and hypofluorescent bands.*

HYPOTONY MACULOPATHY

Definition

Hypotony maculopathy is a condition in which chorioretinal folds develop in the posterior pole of patients with chronically low intraocular pressure.

Epidemiology and Etiology

Patients with chronically low intraocular pressure from a wound leak, cyclodialysis cleft, or excessive filtering after glaucoma surgery may develop secondary retinal changes.

History

Patients will experience loss of central vision from the chorioretinal folds.

Important Clinical Signs

Broad chorioretinal folds radiate out temporally from the optic nerve in a branching fashion (Figure 2-29). Nasally the folds are usually arranged concentric to the optic nerve or have an irregular arrangement. The macular retina may be thrown into radiating folds around the fovea distinct from the choroidal folds. The peripapillary choroid is often swollen, mimicking optic disc edema.

Associated Clinical Signs

The intraocular pressure will be low, usually less than 5 mm Hg. There may be anterior segment signs consistent with surgery or trauma.

Differential Diagnosis

Chorioretinal folds from other causes (see Table 2-3)

Diagnostic Evaluation

Fluorescein angiography will demonstrate alternating hypofluorescent and hyperfluorescent lines corresponding to the folds. Optic disc hyperfluorescence and macular leakage may be observed.

Prognosis and Management

Surgical correction of the underlying cause of hypotony maculopathy will usually result in resolution of the folds and visual improvement. Long-standing folds may resolve with treatment, but there may be residual linear retinal pigment epithelial alterations from the chronic folding of the retinal pigment epithelium.

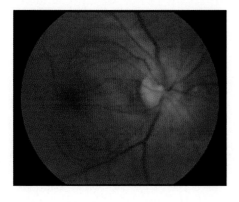

Figure 2-29 Hypotony maculopathy *Horizontal and oblique macular folds in a patient with hypotony maculopathy after glaucoma surgery.*

Chapter 3

DIABETIC RETINOPATHY

James F. Vander, MD

DIABETIC RETINOPATHY

Definition

Diabetic retinopathy encompasses a broad range of fundus manifestations of diabetes mellitus. This is a clinical term that includes exudative, hemorrhagic, ischemic, proliferative, and tractional manifestations of this retinal vascular disease. It can be arbitrarily divided into a nonproliferative and proliferative form.

Epidemiology and Etiology

Incidence   Diabetic retinopathy is the leading cause of blindness in the United States and Western Europe among adults less than age 55 years. It affects both genders and all races, although African Americans are more frequently and more severely affected than Caucasians.

Risk Factor   The best predictor of diabetic retinopathy is the duration of disease. For type 1 diabetic patients there is no risk of retinopathy for roughly 5 years after initial diagnosis. Some retinopathy is present in up to 50% of patients 10 years after diagnosis. After 15 years, 95% of patients show some retinopathy. Proliferative retinopathy is very uncommon with less than 10 years' duration of disease. Forty percent of patients have proliferative disease by 25 years.

The trend for type 2 diabetic patients is very similar. Many patients will have asymptomatic, occult diabetes for many years prior to diagnosis, however, and therefore may present with retinopathy even at the time of diagnosis of diabetes mellitus.

Age is another important risk factor in the prevalence of diabetic retinopathy. Diabetic retinopathy is very rare prior to puberty. Its prevalence increases dramatically after puberty, however, and over 50% of patients will develop retinopathy by their early twenties.

Pathophysiology

Hyperglycemia is a key factor in the development of diabetic retinopathy. The mechanism of retinopathy development may be related to:

Relative hypercoagulability
Red blood cell abnormalities
Excessive glycosylation of proteins
Enzymatic conversion of excessive glucose
    by aldose reductase

Histopathologically, thickening of retinal capillary basement membranes and loss of pericytes have been shown consistently.

History

Patients are often asymptomatic but may have blurry vision or floaters. More extensive visual loss occurs with large vitreous hemorrhages or retinal detachment.

NONPROLIFERATIVE DIABETIC RETINOPATHY

Important Clinical Signs

Nonproliferative retinopathy (NPDR) is the preferred term for this less severe manifestation of diabetic retinopathy. It may be arbitrarily subdivided into mild, moderate, and severe categories.

Mild Nonproliferative Diabetic Retinopathy
Earliest fundus manifestations of diabetic retinopathy. Features reflect retinal capillary hyperpermeability. May be manifest as:

> *Intraretinal hemorrhage*—dot hemorrhages are small mid-level retinal hemorrhages (Figure 3-1A,B).
> *Blot hemorrhages*—larger, with fuzzier borders.
> *Flame-shaped hemorrhages*—superficial in the nerve fiber layer.
> *Microaneurysms*—saccular enlargement of retinal capillaries.
> *Lipoprotein exudation*—also known as hard yellow exudate (Figures 3-2 and 3-3).
> *Macular edema*—the most common reason for legal blindness resulting from diabetic

retinopathy. It is best appreciated as macular thickening by the use of a high magnification slit-lamp examination using a hand held or contact lens providing a good stereoscopic view (Figure 3-4A–D).

Moderate Nonproliferative Diabetic Retinopathy This degree of retinopathy is characterized by increased number and size of intraretinal hemorrhaging with greater evidence for exudation as manifest by more hard yellow exudate (Figure 3-5) and macular edema than is present in mild nonproliferative retinopathy. (Standardized photographs exist to establish the transition points between the various stages of nonproliferative retinopathy, but it should be remembered that this classification reflects a continuum of disease severity.) In moderate nonproliferative retinopathy one also begins to see evidence of capillary occlusive disease. This is reflected by the development of:

Cotton-wool spots (Figure 3-6)
Venous dilation and beading (Figure 3-7)

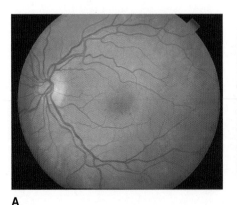
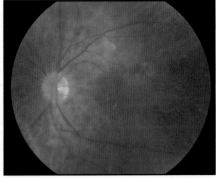

A **B**

Figure 3-1 *A,B. Minimal nonproliferative diabetic retinopathy (NPDR).*

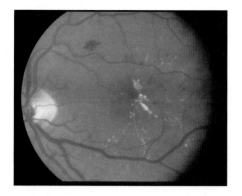

Figure 3-2 *NPDR with retinal hemorrhages and hard yellow exudates (HYE).*

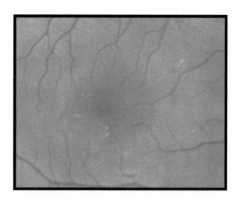

Figure 3-3 *Subtle HYE near fovea in NPDR.*

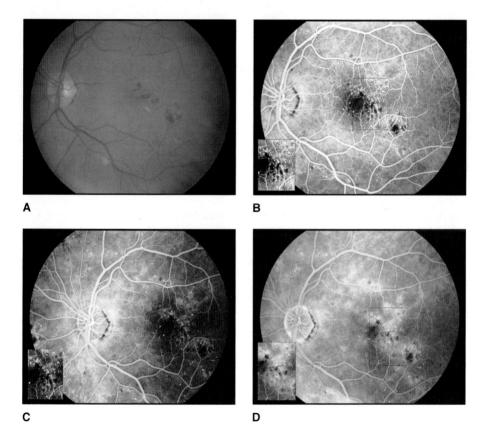

Figure 3-4 *A. Retinal hemorrhages, HYE, and edema in NPDR. B. Venous phase intravenous fluorescein angiogram (IVFA) showing numerous microaneurysms seen as pinpoint dots of hyperfluorescence. C. Leakage from microaneurysms with obscuration of hyperfluorescent dots. D. Later phase showing more extensive leakage.*

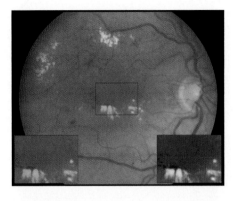

Figure 3-5 *Macular edema and HYE with blunting of foveal reflex* (insets).

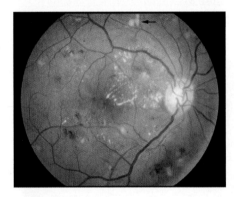

Figure 3-6 *Cotton-wool spots as well as hemorrhage and HYE.*

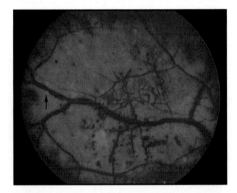

Figure 3-7 *Venous beading* (arrow) *indicating more severe NPDR.*

Intraretinal microvascular abnormality (IRMA)—flat, intraretinal, irregular blood vessel. (It is sometimes difficult to distinguish between IRMA and neovascularization of the retina. Fluorescein angiography can be helpful in making this distinction; see Figure 3-8B.)

Vision loss in moderate NPDR may be the result of macular edema or, less frequently, loss of some of the normal perifoveolar capillary bed. Frequently, both problems may be present.

Severe Nonproliferative Retinopathy In severe NPDR there is worsening of the exudative aspect of diabetic retinopathy and, especially, evidence for capillary occlusive changes. More extensive intraretinal hemorrhaging, venous beading, IRMA, as well as edema and exudate are the features that define severe

nonproliferative retinopathy (Figure 3-8A–C, 3-9, and 3-10). The presence of certain fundus features predicts the progression toward proliferative retinopathy (Table 3-1).

Associated Clinical Signs

Other features associated with NPDR are:

Cornea—decrease of corneal sensitivity; increased risk abrasion

Cataract—typically nuclear and cortical cataract formation is chronic and progressive; acute cortical cataract formation with profound elevations in blood glucose

Glaucoma—greater incidence of primary open-angle glaucoma

Cranial nerve palsy—isolated palsy, most often sixth

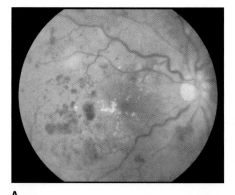

A

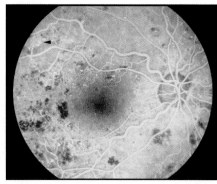

B

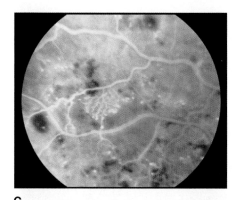

C

Figure 3-8 *A. Severe NPDR.* ***B.*** *IVFA shows numerous microaneurysms and patches of capillary nonperfusion* (arrowhead). *Note abnormal vessels (intraretinal microvascular abnormality; IRMA) along superotemporal arcade (*arrowhead*).* ***C.*** *High-powered view of IRMA seen in (****B****). Absence of leakage distinguishes IRMA from neovascularization.*

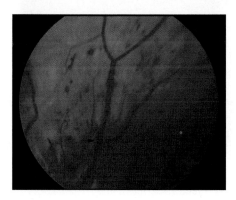

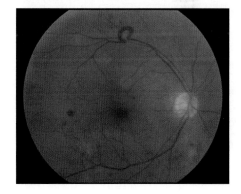

Figure 3-9 *Sausaging of retinal venules* (arrow) *seen in severe NPDR.*

Figure 3-10 *Venous loop.*

TABLE 3-1 4-2-1 RULE

The presence of:
   Severe retinal hemorrhages in **4** quadrants
      or
   Venous beading in **2** quadrants
      or
   IRMA in **1** quadrant
Indicates a 50% risk of developing proliferative retinopathy within 1 year

Differential Diagnosis

Other causes of retinal capillary leakage and occlusion include:

   Hypertensive retinopathy
   Retinal vein occlusion (branch or central) (Figure 3-11)
   Hemoglobinopathies
   Anemia or leukemia
   Ocular ischemic syndrome
   Radiation retinopathy (Figure 3-12)
   Idiopathic juxtafoveal telangiectasis
   Coats' disease
   Vasculitis (e.g., sarcoidosis, lupus)

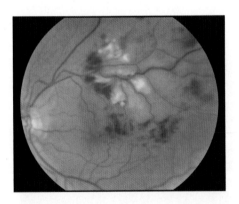

Figure 3-11 *Hemorrhages and cotton-wool spots in branch retinal vein obstruction. Note the segmental distribution of the fundus abnormalities.*

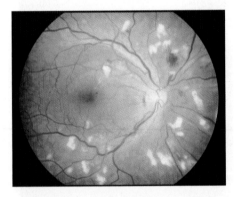

Figure 3-12 *Numerous cotton-wool spots with a few hemorrhages in a nondiabetic patient with a history of prior radiation for treatment of a brain tumor.*

TABLE 3-2 **CLINICALLY SIGNIFICANT MACULAR EDEMA (CSME)**

Retinal thickening within 500 μm center of fovea
or
Exudate within 500 μm center of fovea with adjacent thickening
or
Thickening of at least one disc area any part within one disc diameter of center of fovea

Note: CSME is a diagnosis based on stereoscopic macular viewing independent of visual acuity or fluorescein angiography.

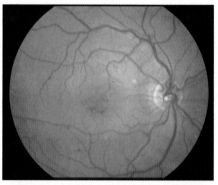

A

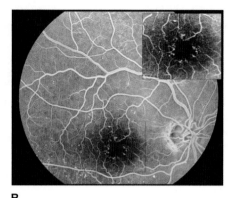

B

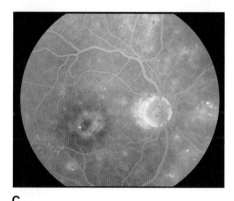

C

Figure 3-13 *A. Retinal hemorrhages with mild macular edema. **B.** Enlargement of the foveal avascular zone with microaneurysms near the center of the macula (inset). **C.** Late leakage from the microaneurysms.*

Diagnostic Evaluation

The most important aspect of the evaluation of NPDR is a magnified, stereoscopic, slit-lamp biomicroscopic examination of the posterior pole and midperipheral retina using a handheld indirect lens or contact lens. A critical determination is the presence or absence of clinically significant macular edema (CSME; Table 3-2).

Fluorescein angiography is a valuable ancillary test in evaluation of NPDR. Indications include:

Determination of location of focal and diffuse leakage to guide treatment (Figure 3-13A–C)
Rule out loss of perifoveal capillaries
Mechanism for unexplained vision loss
Risk factor for vision loss after focal laser
Rule out vasculitis or other diagnostic possibilities

Prognosis and Management

Nonproliferative diabetic retinopathy tends to progress gradually over months to years. The risk of vision loss increases with increasing severity of retinopathy. Treatment of systemic disease reduces but does not eliminate the risk of progression and vision loss (Table 3-3). Newer medications under development may actually reverse retinopathy.

Ocular treatment consists of macular laser photocoagulation for macular edema (Figure 3-14A–B). Early Treatment Diabetic Retinopathy Study (ETDRS) guidelines are widely applied (see Table 3-4; see also Appendix Table A-8). The utility and timing of retreatment, the role of early treatment before ETDRS threshold is reached, and the application of alternative treatment strategies are less uniformly accepted (Table 3-4).

The ETDRS addressed three questions:

1. What is the role of aspirin in diabetic retinopathy? *Answer:* It neither improves nor worsens retinopathy.
2. What is the role of initiating early laser (as compared to DRS high-risk criteria; see Table 3-5) in the management of severe nonproliferative and early proliferative retinopathy? *Answer:* Inconclusive. No strong benefit to early scatter panretinal photocoagulation (PRP) was found. Certain clinical circumstances (e.g., poor compliance with follow-up examinations, rapid progression in fellow eye) may justify early initiation of PRP.
3. What is the role of laser (PRP or focal macular laser, or both) in the management of macular edema? *Answer:* There is no role for PRP in treatment of macular edema. Macular laser is of benefit, reducing the risk of moderate visual loss by 50%. Patients with CSME should be treated.

TABLE 3-3 DIABETES CONTROL AND COMPLICATIONS TRIAL (DCCT)

DCCT showed that tightened blood glucose control reduces:
 Development of retinopathy by 76%
 Progression of retinopathy by 80%
 Risk of nephropathy by about 60%
 Risk of neuropathy by about 60%

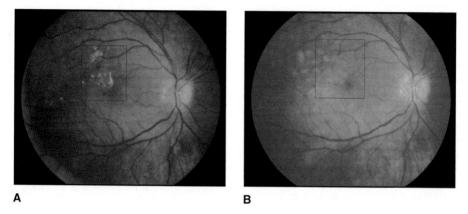

A   **B**

Figure 3-14 *A. Macular edema and HYE in NPDR. **B.** Several months after laser treatment, resolution of edema and HYE is seen.*

TABLE 3-4 EARLY TREATMENT DIABETIC RETINOPATHY STUDY (ETDRS) FACTS

ETDRS treatment of macular edema:

    Generally stabilizes visual acuity but often does not improve it

    Consists of directly treating focal areas of leakage and placing a grid in areas of diffuse capillary leakage; determination of treatment placement is generally guided by the use of a fluorescein angiogram

    Should be avoided in presence of significant loss of perifoveal capillaries

    May take months to show resolution of thickening and longer for exudates

PROLIFERATIVE DIABETIC RETINOPATHY

Proliferative diabetic retinopathy (PDR) represents the most severe manifestation of diabetes in the eye. It is the result of the loss of normal retinal perfusion and the subsequent development of neovascular proliferative tissue in the fundus. The development of this neovascular tissue reflects an alteration in the balance between angiogenesis inhibitors and stimulators in the retina and vitreous. Multiple local chemical mediators (cytokines) are believed to be at work.

Important Clinical Signs

Neovascularization of the Disc (NVD) Neovascularization that develops on the surface of the optic nerve or within one disc diameter of the optic nerve is defined as NVD (Figures 3-15, 3-16, and 3-17A–D; see also Figure 3-19A–D). Shunt vessels that may develop on the optic disc (e.g., after a retinal venous obstruction) may be easily confused with NVD. Neovascularization of the disc typically has a lacy irregular appearance and may be elevated above the optic nerve surface. True NVD should be distinguished from the hyperemic disc swelling of diabetic papillopathy.

Neovascularization Elsewhere (NVE) This term refers to retinal neovascularization anywhere in the fundus that is not NVD (Figures 3-18A–D and 3-19A–D). Neovascularization elsewhere in PDR tends to occur in the posterior pole or midperiphery, although extreme peripheral NVE can also develop. Neovascularization elsewhere tends to form at the junction between perfused and nonperfused retina, and this can be readily appreciated with fluorescein angiography.

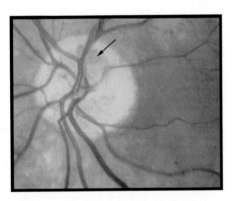

Figure 3-15 Neovascularization of the disc (NVD) *Moderately severe NVD as defined in the Diabetic Retinopathy Study. (Standard Photo 10A, courtesy of the Diabetic Retinopathy Study Group.)*

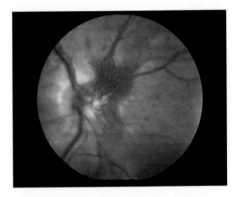

Figure 3-16 *Severe elevated NVD.*

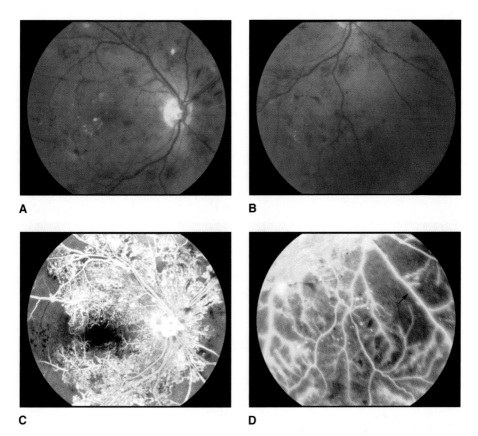

Figure 3-17 *A. Proliferative diabetic retinopathy (PDR) with macular edema, HYE, and NVD. B. View of the inferior midperiphery with some hemorrhages and a bland fundus appearance. C. IVFA confirming NVD and showing profound occlusion of large and small retinal vessels. D. IVFA of inferior fundus showing severe capillary occlusion and ischemic staining of the large vessel walls* (arrow).

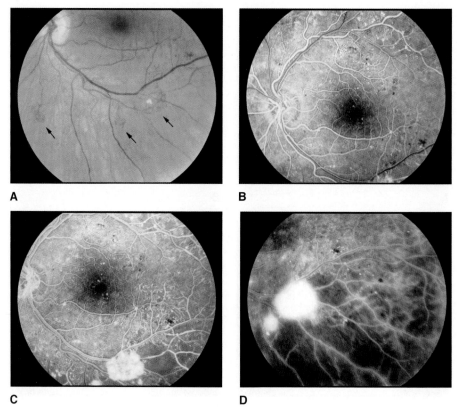

Figure 3-18 *A. Patches of neovascularization elsewhere (NVE). Note the bland appearance of the fundus peripheral to the NVE. **B**. Macular view on IVFA demonstrates microaneurysms but minimal ischemia. **C**. Hyperfluorescence of the NVE. **D**. Note the marked capillary nonperfusion peripheral to the NVE.*

Neovascularization of the Iris (NVI) Development of NVI is an ominous sign (Figure 3-20). Involvement of the anterior chamber angle can produce neovascular glaucoma (NVG), leading to a blind, painful eye.

Vitreous Hemorrhage Bleeding from NVD or NVE may occur and produce preretinal or vitreous hemorrhage. Vitreous hemorrhage is more likely when NVD and NVE are more extensive. Hemorrhages are usually spontaneous and produce a sudden development of floaters. Preretinal hemorrhage reflects sequestration of blood between the inner retinal surface and an intact posterior hyaloid face (Figure 3-21). Therefore, this will generally occur in younger patients. This may produce a dense, well-circumscribed scotoma (Figures 3-22 and 3-25A–D). Often preretinal hemorrhage will subsequently break apart and produce more diffuse floaters characteristic of vitreous hemorrhage (Figures 3-23 and 3-24). Vitreous hemorrhage is often recurrent and can produce profound visual loss.

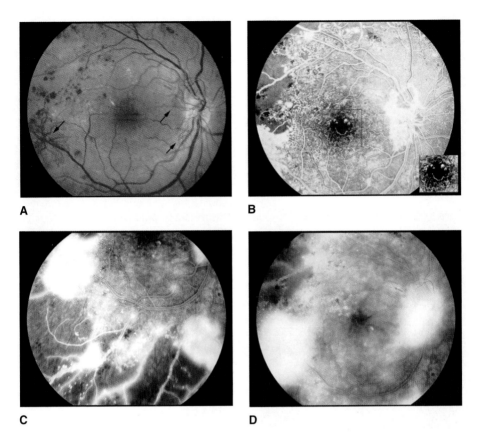

Figure 3-19 *A. PDR with NVD and NVE (arrows). **B.** IVFA showing hyperfluorescence of NVD and NVE. Note the irregular capillary bed in the central macula (inset). **C.** Marked hyperfluorescence of NVE with peripheral nonperfusion. **D.** Marked late hyperfluorescence from leaking NVD and NVE with macular edema.*

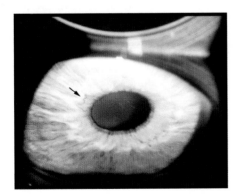

Figure 3-20 *Neovascularization of the iris in PDR seen through a gonioscopic mirror.*

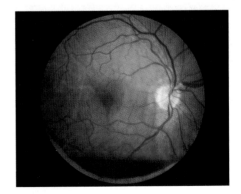

Figure 3-21 *Boat-shaped preretinal hemorrhage in PDR.*

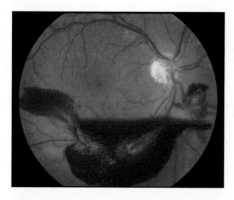

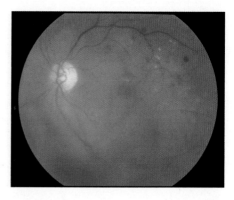

Figure 3-22 *Large preretinal hemorrhage in PDR resulting in a large, dense scotoma.*

Figure 3-23 *Mild vitreous hemorrhage in PDR.*

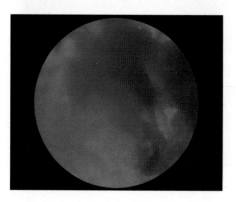

Figure 3-24 *More dense vitreous hemorrhage.*

TABLE 3-5 DIABETIC RETINOPATHY STUDY (DRS)

DRS showed:
  Risk features for severe visual loss (defined as visual acuity of 5/200 or worse) are:
  NVD > ⅓ to ¼ of disc area
  Any NVD with associated VH
  NVE with associated VH
These features are known as **high-risk characteristics** (HRC). Patients with HRC treated with
  PRP have a 50% reduction in risk of severe visual loss.

NVD = neovascularization of the disc; NVE = neovascularization elsewhere; PRP = panretinal photocoagulation;
    VH = vitreous hemorrhage.

TABLE 3-6 PANRETINAL PHOTOCOAGULATION (PRP) FACTS

PRP:
  Does not improve visual acuity
  May cause worsening macular edema, and loss of peripheral vision and night vision
  Indications for supplementation are uncertain
  Does not always cause regression of NVD/NVE
  Is also indicated in patients with NVI from PDR even in the absence of NVD/NVE

NVD = neovascularization of the disc; NVE = neovascularization elsewhere; NVI = neovascularization of the iris;
    PDR = proliferative diabetic retinopathy.

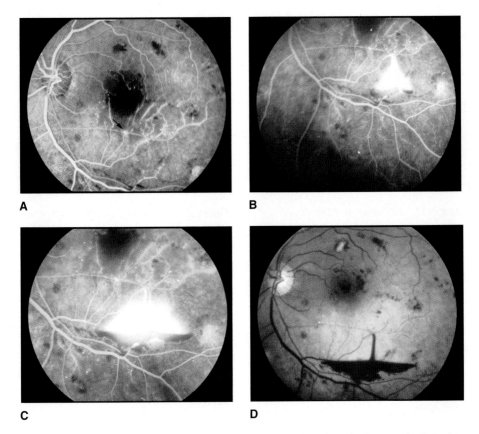

A   B

C   D

Figure 3-25 *A. Early-phase IVFA showing enlargement of foveal avascular zone in diabetic retinopathy. Note the hyperfluorescent dot inferior to the fovea* (arrow). *B. Hyperfluorescence and linear horizontal hypofluorescence develop suddenly during the IVFA as spontaneous preretinal hemorrhage begins to occur from a tiny area of NVE. C. The area of hyper- and hypofluorescence enlarges as hemorrhage expands during the IVFA. D. Red-free photograph showing fresh preretinal hemorrhage. Photo was taken shortly after (C).*

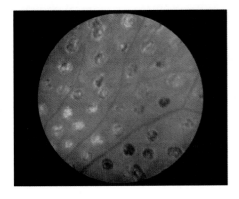

Figure 3-26 *Laser photocoagulation scars spaced about one burn width apart in panretinal photocoagulation (PRP).*

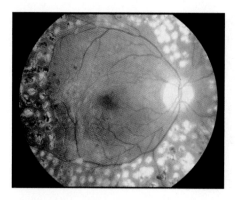

Figure 3-27 *PRP scars in PDR. Note sparing of the macula.*

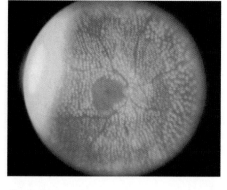

Figure 3-28 *Equator-plus photo after full PRP.*

Management

The treatment of proliferative retinopathy is guided by the Diabetic Retinopathy Study (DRS; Tables 3-5 and 3-6). Laser PRP as established by the DRS is the treatment of choice (Figures 3-26 through 3-28). For eyes with more advanced nonclearing vitreous hemorrhage or fibrovascular scarring, or both, vitrectomy may be indicated.

Macular Ischemia There is no effective treatment for diabetic macular ischemia. This condition more commonly occurs in eyes with proliferative diabetic retinopathy but may be observed in association with nonproliferative disease as well. Irregular enlargement of the foveal avascular zone on fluorescein angiography is observed (Figure 3-29A–D).

Retinal Detachment The development of neovascular tissue produces an unusually strong adhesion between the vitreous and retina. With contraction of the vitreous as well as the fibrovascular proliferative tissue, increasing traction on the retina will develop. Sufficient traction may ultimately lead to a retinal detachment. A traction retinal detachment typically has a concave, immobile appearance with retinal striae radiating from the areas of greatest traction.

When traction retinal detachment affects the macula, severe visual loss is noted.

Combined traction and rhegmatogenous retinal detachment may develop if vitreous traction is severe enough to produce a full-thickness retinal break. Combined retinal detachments tend to develop more rapidly than purely tractional retinal detachments. The retina appears more mobile with corrugations and undulations noted with eye movement.

Indications for Vitrectomy in Proliferative Diabetic Retinopathy

DEFINITE

Persistent or recurrent vitreous hemorrhage (Figure 3-30A,B)

Traction macular detachment (Figures 3-31A,B and 3-32A,B)

Combined traction and rhegmatogenous retinal detachment (Figure 3-33)

POSSIBLE

Severe proliferation unresponsive to PRP

Traction detachment threatening the macula

Persistent macular edema with taut posterior hyaloid face

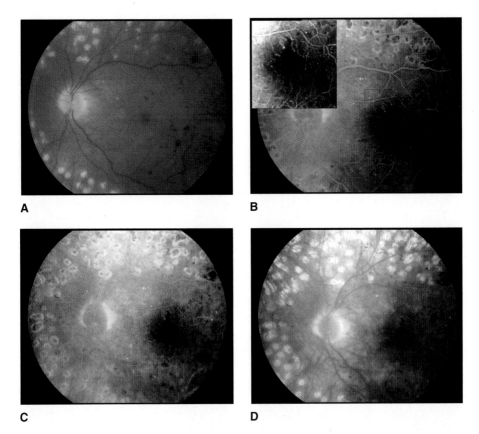

A

B

C

D

Figure 3-29 *A. Posterior pole after PRP. The patient had no appreciable macular thickening but vision was reduced to 20/80. **B–D.** IVFA showing enlarged, irregular foveal avascular zone (**B,** inset) identifying ischemia as the mechanism of vision loss.*

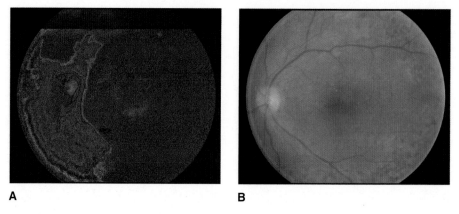

Figure 3-30 *A. Large premacular hemorrhage with marked vision loss. **B.** Appearance after vitrectomy and PRP.*

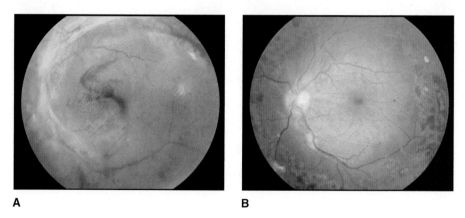

Figure 3-31 *A. Traction retinal detachment involving the macula. **B.** Postoperative appearance after vitrectomy, membrane peeling, and PRP.*

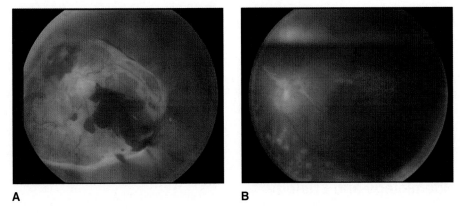

Figure 3-32A,B *A. Marked traction on the macula in a patient found to have a full-thickness retinal break as well during vitrectomy. **B.** Postoperative appearance shows the retina to be attached, PRP and a residual vitreous cavity gas bubble* (arrow) *slowly resolving.*

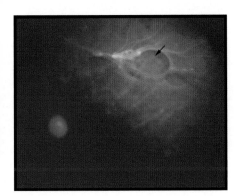

Figure 3-33 *Combined traction and rhegmatogenous retinal disease in PDR. Note the full-thickness retinal hole* (arrow) *and adjacent white fibrovascular traction on the elevated retinal vessel.*

DIABETIC PAPILLOPATHY

Definition

Diabetic papillopathy describes optic disc edema, either unilateral or bilateral, in a diabetic patient with evidence for minimal or mild optic nerve dysfunction and no evidence for ocular inflammation or elevated intracranial pressure.

Epidemiology and Etiology

Roughly 70% of patients have type 1 diabetes, and 60% of cases are unilateral. Etiology is uncertain, although some suggest a mild non-arteritic ischemic optic neuropathy (AION).

History

Patients may have blurry vision or be asymptomatic. Rarely there will be transient visual obscuration. Neurologic symptoms are absent.

Important Clinical Signs

Disc swelling occurs with prominent surface vessels and fine hemorrhages on the disc (Figure 3-34A,B). An afferent papillary defect is present but generally not severe. Visual loss is often mild with 20/40 or better in 75% of cases.

Associated Clinical Signs

A crowded optic disc is often present similar to AION. This does not correlate with the degree of diabetic retinopathy.

Differential Diagnosis

> Optic disc neovascularization from PDR
> AION
> Optic neuritis
> Optic disc drusen
> Papilledema

Diagnostic Evaluation

In general, no workup is needed in the appropriate clinical setting. If the case is atypical, then imaging such as a magnetic resonance scan is

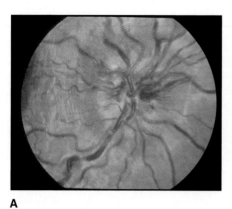
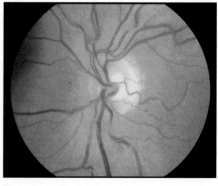

A **B**

Figure 3-34 *A. Disc edema with hemorrhages in diabetic papillopathy. **B.** Fellow eye shows a normal optic nerve and no appreciable diabetic retinopathy.*

CHAPTER 3. DIABETIC RETINOPATHY

indicated. Visual field examination may be useful to document and follow visual loss. Fluorescein angiography can distinguish diabetic papillopathy from NVD but is rarely needed. Diabetic papillopathy (Figure 3-35A–C) typically stains without significant leakage on fluorescein angiography whereas NVD shows leakage of dye into the vitreous cavity.

Prognosis and Management

No treatment is indicated. Substantial spontaneous recovery occurs, usually over weeks to months, with many patients showing subtle optic atrophy or visual field defects permanently. Patients should be monitored to rule out rapid progression to proliferative diabetic retinopathy, which occurs in a minority of cases.

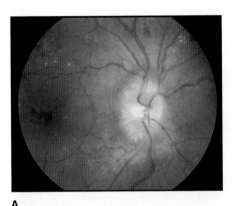

A

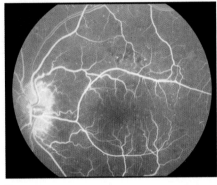

B

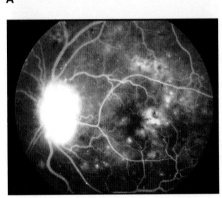

C

Figure 3-35 *A. Diabetic papillopathy with disc swelling as well as scattered retinal hemorrhages and HYE. **B.** Disc hyperfluorescence with a few retinal microaneurysms. **C.** Marked staining of the optic disc but no significant leakage of dye into the vitreous cavity.*

Chapter 4

RETINAL VASCULAR DISEASE

Gary C. Brown, MD

COTTON-WOOL SPOTS

Definition

Cotton-wool spots describe the retinal change resulting from acute blockage of blood flow within a terminal retinal arteriole.

Epidemiology and Etiology

The prevalence is uncertain. Cotton-wool spots are seen in over 40% of cases of diabetic retinopathy and also with acute systemic arterial hypertension. No hereditary pattern is known.

Pathophysiology

Embolic
Hypertensive arteriolar necrosis
Inflammatory
See "Diagnostic Evaluation" on opposite page

Clinical Signs

Visual Acuity Central visual acuity is usually unaffected, although patients may note the sudden appearance of corresponding blind spots.

Pupillary Changes An afferent pupillary defect is usually absent.

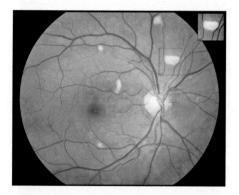

Figure 4-1 Cotton-wool spots *Multiple cotton-wool spots* (inset) *in the fundus of a patient with human immunodeficiency virus (HIV) infection.*

Fundus Changes Cotton-wool spots appear in the posterior pole of the fundus (not the peripheral retina) as superficial areas of retinal opacification that characteristically measure less than one quarter disc area in size (Figure 4-1). When associated with diabetes mellitus, systemic arterial hypertension, and retinal venous obstruction, they are generally seen concomitantly with retinal hemorrhages. Cotton-wool spots usually resolve over 5 to 7 weeks but may remain longer when present in conjunction with diabetic retinopathy.

Differential Diagnosis

Inflammatory retinitis may occur from entities such as toxoplasmosis or cytomegalovirus. Retinal hemorrhages are typically present with the latter. There are also usually vitreous cells present with inflammatory conditions, but not with cotton-wool spots alone.

Diagnostic Evaluation

Intravenous fluorescein angiography is minimally helpful. It reveals areas of relative hypofluorescence corresponding to the cotton-wool spots.

Systemic workup (similar to that of acute central retinal artery obstruction, unless the obvious causes of diabetic retinopathy, systemic arterial hypertension, and retinal venous obstruction are present):

Diabetic retinopathy—cotton-wool spots are present in 44% of cases.
Systemic arterial hypertension—diastolic blood pressure of 110 to 115 mm Hg or more is usually necessary to induce cotton-wool spot formation in adults.
Retinal vein obstruction—central, branch.
Embolic—carotid and cardiac.
Inflammatory—giant cell arteritis, Wegener's granulomatosis, polyarteritis nodosa, systemic lupus erythematosus, scleroderma, orbital mucormycosis, toxoplasmosis retinitis.

Coagulopathies—sickle cell disease, homocysteinuria, lupus anticoagulant syndrome, protein S deficiency, protein C deficiency, antithrombin III deficiency.
Miscellaneous—migraine, Lyme disease, hypotension, acquired immunodeficiency syndrome (AIDS), interferon therapy, metastatic carcinoma, intravenous drug abuse (chronic), papilledema, acute pancreatitis, severe anemia, radiation retinopathy, leptospirosis, Purtscher's retinopathy.

Prognosis and Management

The visual prognosis for central vision is good unless there are innumerable cotton-wool spots as with entities such as systemic lupus erythematosus, pancreatitis, Purtcher's retinopathy, or intravenous drug abuse. Associated damage from entities that cotton-wool spots accompany (e.g., diabetic retinopathy or retinal venous obstruction) can lead to severe visual loss.

There is no consistently proven treatment to ameliorate the visual acuity. When diabetic retinopathy and retinal vein obstruction are excluded as causes, a serious associated systemic disease can be found in 95% of cases. Thus, it is critical to undertake a systemic workup if there is no appreciable underlying cause, even if only one cotton-wool spot is present.

HYPERTENSIVE RETINOPATHY

Definition

Hypertensive retinopathy refers to the retinal vascular changes associated with systemic arterial hypertension. Hypertensive choroidopathy may also accompany the acute phases of hypertensive retinopathy.

Epidemiology

Hypertensive retinopathy can be divided into chronic and acute phases. The most commonly used classification is the Keith-Wagener-Barker classification. The grades of hypertensive retinopathy are as follows:

> *Grade 1*—retinal arterial narrowing (Figure 4-2)
>
> *Grade 2*—retinal arteriovenous nicking (Figure 4-3)
>
> *Grade 3*—retinal hemorrhages, cotton-wool spots, hard exudates (Figure 4-4)
>
> *Grade 4*—grade 3 changes plus optic disc swelling (Figure 4-5A–C)

Grades 1 and 2 are commonly seen in practice. Grade 3 and 4 changes are much less frequently seen.

Pathophysiology

Grades 1 and 2 Hyalinization and thickening of the retinal arterial walls is seen, leading to the straightened vessels in grade 1 and the indentation (nicking) of the retinal veins by the arteries in grade 2 hypertensive retinopathy.

Grade 3 The systemic diastolic blood pressure in an adult with grade 3 hypertensive retinopathy is typically at least 110 to 115 mm Hg. At this point, the retinal arteries lose their ability to autoregulate the blood flow, and the high pressure is passed distally to the retinal arterioles and capillary bed.

Grade 4 The systemic diastolic blood pressure in an adult with grade 4 hypertensive retinopathy is usually at least 130 to 140 mm Hg. With both grades 3 and 4 hypertensive retinopathy, the increased blood pressure can damage the blood vessel wall, leading to fibrinoid necrosis (the presence of fibrin thrombi within the vascular lumina). A similar process occurs with hypertensive choroidopathy, leading to necrosis of the overlying retinal pigment epithelium (Elschnig spot).

Clinical Signs

Grade 1 and 2 changes are chronic, whereas grade 3 and 4 changes indicate acute retinal vascular decompensation. Hypertensive choroidopathy (Elschnig spots) may accompany grade 3 and 4 changes. Elschnig spots are round and yellow acutely, eventually changing to pigmented lesions.

Differential Diagnosis

Diabetic retinopathy, radiation retinopathy, venous occlusive disease, carotid artery occlusive disease (ocular ischemic syndrome), and collagen vascular diseases can all mimic the changes of hypertensive retinopathy.

Diagnostic Evaluation

Measurement of the systemic blood pressure is critical when the diagnosis is suspected. If the acute changes (grades 3 and 4) are classic and the blood pressure is not elevated at the time of measurement, consideration should be given to the possibility the blood pressure has been uncontrolled recently or is uncontrolled at other times during the day.

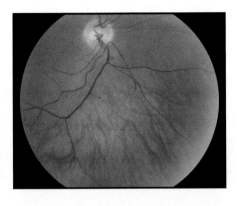

Figure 4-2 Hypertensive retinopathy, grade 1 *The retinal arteries are markedly narrowed and straightened. Small retinal hemorrhages are present, due not to hypertension but to background diabetic retinopathy.*

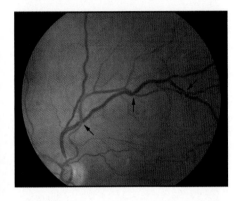

Figure 4-3 Hypertensive retinopathy, grade 2 *Prominent arteriovenous nicking (arrows) is seen. Small retinal hemorrhages are present, due not to hypertension, but to diabetic retinopathy.*

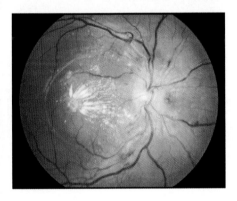

Figure 4-4 Hypertensive retinopathy, grade 3 *Cotton-wool spots, retinal hemorrhages, a macular star composed of intraretinal lipid exudates, and a serous detachment of the macula are all present.*

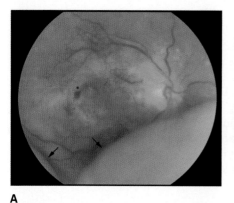

A

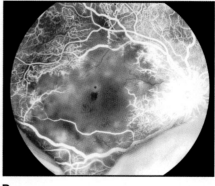

B

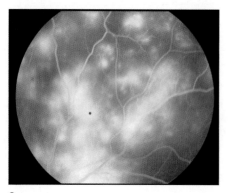

C

Figure 4-5   Hypertensive retinopathy, grade 4   *A. Retinal hemorrhages are present, the optic disc is swollen, and an exudative retinal detachment* (arrows) *is present inferiorly. Yellow Elschnig spots* (asterisk) *are present in the macula. B. Fluorescein angiogram corresponding to (A). Profound retinal capillary nonperfusion is present in the macula (macular ischemia), and foci of hyperfluorescence corresponding to the Elschnig spots* (asterisk) *are also seen in the macula. C. Fluorescein angiogram of the superior fundus of the eye shown in (A). Numerous foci of hyperfluorescence corresponding to Elschnig spots* (asterisk) *can be seen.*

Prognosis and Management

Vision is typically unaffected with grades 1 and 2 hypertensive retinopathy and may be mildly decreased with grade 3 retinopathy. With grade 4 retinopathy, vision can be markedly decreased due to retinal edema, hard exudates in the central macula (macular star), or the presence of a serous retinal detachment.

The treatment for hypertensive retinopathy is to correct the underlying condition by normalizing the blood pressure. This causes resolution of the fundus abnormalities over a period of weeks to months in eyes with grade 3 and 4 changes, but often does not affect the changes seen with grades 1 and 2 hypertensive retinopathy.

Laser therapy has not been shown to be of benefit in treating the visual loss associated with grades 3 and 4 hypertensive retinopathy. Correcting the blood pressure after grade 4 retinopathy can lead to visual improvement, although there may be some residual, permanent visual loss.

CILIORETINAL ARTERY OBSTRUCTION (OCCLUSION)

Definition

This entity describes the acute blockage of blood flow within a cilioretinal artery.

Epidemiology and Etiology

Cilioretinal artery obstruction typically occurs in patients aged 65 years and older but can be seen at any age. It is seen in approximately 1:100,000 outpatient ophthalmology visits. The abnormality is unilateral in over 99% of cases. No hereditary pattern is known.

Pathophysiology

Embolic
Hypertensive arterial necrosis
Inflammatory (e.g., giant cell arteritis)
Hemorrhage under an atherosclerotic plaque
Associated with central retinal vein obstruction

Clinical Signs

Visual Acuity Generally, there is a history of acute, unilateral, painless visual field loss occurring over several seconds. Approximately 10% of those affected have a history of transient visual loss (amaurosis fugax) in the affected eye.

Pupillary Changes An afferent pupillary defect may present immediately, depending on the area of distribution of the obstruction.

Fundus Changes Three variants occur:

1. *Cilioretinal artery obstruction alone* (Figure 4-6)—superficial retinal whitening, usually located within the papillomacular bundle, which may take hours to develop
2. *Cilioretinal artery obstruction associated with central retinal vein obstruction*
3. *Cilioretinal artery obstruction associated with acute anterior ischemic optic neuropathy* (Figure 4-7)—must be particularly concerned about underlying giant cell arteritis

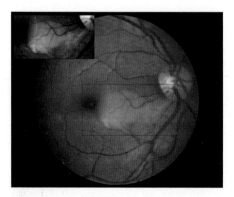

Figure 4-6 Cilioretinal artery obstruction *Isolated cilioretinal artery obstruction. Note the retinal whitening indicating ischemic retinal edema* (inset).

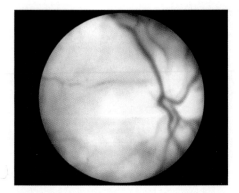

Figure 4-7 Cilioretinal artery obstruction and ischemic optic neuropathy *Cilioretinal artery occlusion associated with anterior ischemic optic neuropathy. Note the associated disc edema and pallor.*

Retinal Intra-arterial Emboli Prevalence is uncertain:

Cholesterol (Hollenhorst plaque)—glistening yellow and typically from the carotid arteries

Calcific—large, white plaque generally originating from the cardiac valves

Fibrin-platelet—longer and dull white; may originate from the carotids or cardiac valves

Differential Diagnosis

Inflammatory retinitis from entities such as toxoplasmosis or cytomegalovirus. Retinal hemorrhages are typically present with the latter. There are also usually vitreous cells present with inflammatory conditions, but not with acute cilioretinal artery obstruction.

Diagnostic Evaluation

Intravenous Fluorescein Angiography
Cilioretinal arteries normally fill with fluorescein dye during the early choroidal filling phase of a fluorescein angiogram. A cilioretinal artery obstruction typically shows nonperfusion of dye in the affected vessel through the retinal arteriovenous phase.

Systemic Workup (This is similar to that of acute central retinal artery obstruction.)

Emboli—carotid and cardiac

Inflammatory—giant cell arteritis, Wegener's granulomatosis, polyarteritis nodosa, systemic lupus erythematosus, orbital mucormycosis, toxoplasmosis retinitis

Coagulopathies—sickle cell disease, homocysteinuria, lupus anticoagulant syndrome, protein S deficiency, protein C deficiency, antithrombin III deficiency

Miscellaneous—fibromuscular hyperplasia, Sydenham's chorea, Fabry's disease, migraine, Lyme disease, hypotension

Prognosis and Management

With isolated cilioretinal artery obstruction, 90% of eyes return to 20/40 vision or better. With central retinal vein occlusion, 70% of eyes return to 20/40 vision or better. With anterior ischemic optic neuropathy, vision often remains counting fingers to hand motions.

There is no consistently proven treatment to ameliorate the visual acuity. Because of the relatively good prognosis for central vision, digital massage and anterior chamber paracentesis are not typically undertaken.

Despite the lack of an effective ocular treatment, a systemic workup should be undertaken. Although giant cell arteritis likely only accounts for 1% to 2% of cases, the possibility should be actively investigated because the fellow eye can be involved by retinal arterial obstruction within hours to days.

BRANCH RETINAL ARTERY OBSTRUCTION (OCCLUSION)

Definition

This entity describes the acute blockage of blood flow within a branch retinal artery.

Epidemiology and Etiology

Branch retinal artery obstruction typically occurs in patients aged 65 years and older but can be seen at any age. It is seen in approximately 1:15,000 to 20,000 outpatient ophthalmology visits. The abnormality is unilateral in 99% of cases. No hereditary pattern is known.

Pathophysiology

Embolic
Hypertensive arterial necrosis
Inflammatory (e.g., giant cell arteritis)
Hemorrhage under an atherosclerotic plaque

Clinical Signs

Visual Acuity Generally, there is a history of acute, unilateral, painless visual field loss occurring over several seconds. Approximately 10% of those affected have a history of transient visual loss (amaurosis fugax) in the affected eye.

Pupillary Changes An afferent pupillary defect may present immediately, depending on the area of distribution of the obstruction.

Fundus Changes Superficial retinal whitening (Figure 4-8A) can take hours to develop. Retinal intra-arterial emboli (prevalence uncertain):

> *Cholesterol (Hollenhorst plaque)*—glistening yellow and typically from the carotid arteries

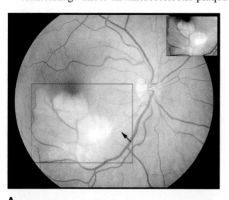

A

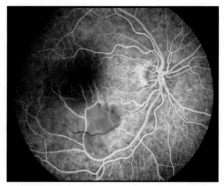

B

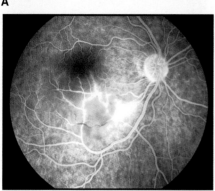

C

Figure 4-8 Branch retinal artery obstruction *A. Retinal whitening* (inset) *due to branch retinal artery obstruction. Note the proximal intra-arterial platelet fibrin thrombus* (arrow). *B. Fluorescein angiogram corresponding to* (*A*) *reveals retinal arteriolar and capillary nonperfusion in the distribution of the occluded vessel. C. Staining of the inferotemporal branch retinal artery is present in the area of occlusion.*

Calcific—large, white plaque generally originating from the cardiac valves (Figure 4-9)

Fibrin-platelet—longer and dull white; may originate from the carotids or cardiac valves (see Figure 4-8A)

Differential Diagnosis

Inflammatory retinitis may occur from entities such as toxoplasmosis or cytomegalovirus. Retinal hemorrhages are typically present with the latter. There are also usually vitreous cells present with inflammatory conditions, but not with acute branch retinal artery obstruction.

Diagnostic Evaluation

Intravenous Fluorescein Angiography
Reveals a delay in retinal arterial and venous filling in the area of obstruction versus the normal remaining fundus (Figure 4-8A,B). There may be staining of the ischemic retinal vasculature (Figure 4-8C).

Systemic Workup   (This is similar to that of acute central retinal artery obstruction.)

Embolic—carotid and cardiac

Inflammatory—giant cell arteritis, Wegener's granulomatosis, polyarteritis nodosa, systemic lupus erythematosus, orbital mucormycosis, toxoplasmosis retinitis

Coagulopathies—sickle cell disease, homocysteinuria, lupus anticoagulant syndrome, protein S deficiency, protein C deficiency, antithrombin III deficiency

Miscellaneous—fibromuscular hyperplasia, Sydenham's chorea, Fabry's disease, migraine, Lyme disease, hypotension

Prognosis and Management

Most patients improve to 20/40 or better vision without treatment, although a field defect corresponding to the area of obstruction usually persists.

There is no consistently proven treatment to ameliorate the visual acuity. Because of the relatively good prognosis for central vision, digital massage and anterior chamber paracentesis are not typically undertaken.

Despite the lack of an effective ocular treatment, a systemic workup should be undertaken. Although giant cell arteritis likely only accounts for 1% to 2% of cases, the possibility should be actively investigated because the fellow eye can be involved within hours to days.

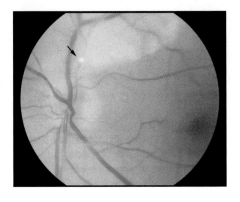

Figure 4-9   Branch retinal artery obstruction, calcific plaque *Intra-arterial calcific plaque* (arrow) *associated with branch retinal artery occlusion.*

CENTRAL RETINAL ARTERY OBSTRUCTION (OCCLUSION)

Definition

This entity describes the acute blockage of blood flow within the central retinal artery.

Epidemiology and Etiology

Central retinal artery obstruction typically occurs in patients aged 65 years and older but can be seen at any age. It is seen in approximately 1:10,000 outpatient ophthalmology visits. The abnormality is unilateral in 99% of cases. No hereditary pattern is known.

Pathophysiology

Embolic
Hypertensive arterial necrosis
Dissecting aneurysm within the central retinal artery
Inflammatory (e.g., giant cell arteritis)
Hemorrhage under an atherosclerotic plaque
Vasospasm

Clinical Signs

Visual Acuity Generally, there is a history of acute, unilateral, painless visual loss occurring over several seconds. Approximately 10% of those affected have a history of transient visual loss (amaurosis fugax) in the affected eye.

Pupillary Changes An afferent pupillary defect is usually present immediately.

Fundus Changes

Superficial retinal whitening—can take hours to develop
Cherry red spot in the foveola (Figure 4-10)
Cilioretinal arterial sparing of central fovea (Figure 4-11)—present in 10% of cases
Retinal intra-arterial emboli—present in 20% of cases
Cholesterol (Hollenhorst plaque)—glistening yellow (Figure 4-12) and typically originates from the carotid arteries
Calcific—large, white plaque generally originating from the cardiac valves
Fibrin-platelet—longer and dull white; may originate from the carotids or cardiac valves (see Figure 4-8A)

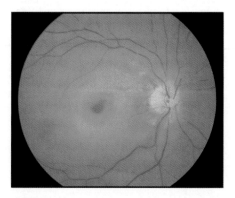

Figure 4-10   Acute central retinal artery occlusion *Superficial retinal opacification is present, and a cherry red spot can be seen in the foveola. Note the segmented columns of blood in retinal arterioles (boxcarring).*

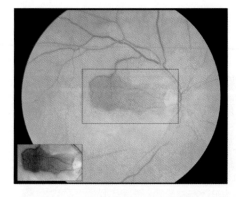

Figure 4-11   Central retinal artery occlusion with cilioretinal artery sparing *Acute central retinal artery occlusion (inset) with cilioretinal arterial sparing of the foveola. Compare with **Figure 4-6**.*

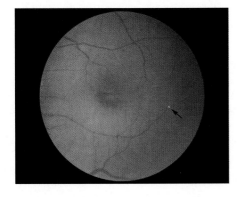

Figure 4-12 Hollenhorst plaque *Glistening cholesterol embolus (Hollenhorst plaque) within a retinal arteriole* (arrow). *These emboli typically lodge at retinal arteriolar bifurcations.*

Differential Diagnosis

Acute ophthalmic artery obstruction (cherry red spot absent)

Tay-Sach's disease (cherry red spot present, but in infants less than 1 year of age and with severe neurologic dysfunction)

Diagnostic Evaluation

Intravenous Fluorescein Angiography Reveals delay in retinal arterial and venous filling (normally, the vein of the temporal vascular arcade should completely fill within 11 seconds after dye enters the corresponding retinal arteries.

Electroretinography Normal a-wave amplitude, but diminished b-wave amplitude.

Systemic Workup

Embolic—carotid and cardiac

Inflammatory—giant cell arteritis, Wegener's granulomatosis, polyarteritis nodosa, systemic lupus erythematosus, orbital mucormycosis

Coagulopathies—sickle cell disease, homocysteinuria, lupus anticoagulant syndrome, protein S deficiency, protein C deficiency, antithrombin III deficiency

Miscellaneous—fibromuscular hyperplasia, Sydenham's chorea, Fabry's disease, migraine, Lyme disease, hypotension

Vasospastic—migraine

Prognosis and Management

The visual prognosis is typically poor, with most patients retaining counting finger to hand motions vision and a small temporal island of vision remaining. If a cilioretinal artery spares the central fovea, 80% of eyes will return to 20/20 to 20/50 vision over a period of 2 weeks. Nevertheless, in the latter instance there is typically severe visual field loss. Approximately 18% of eyes will progress to develop iris neovascularization within 4 to 6 weeks after the acute obstruction.

There is no consistently proven treatment to ameliorate the visual acuity. Digital massage of the globe and anterior chamber paracentesis has been advocated but have minimal benefit. Treatment with fibrinolytic agents is still considered investigational.

Despite the lack of an effective ocular treatment, a systemic workup should be undertaken. Although giant cell arteritis likely only accounts for 1% to 2% of cases, the possibility should be actively investigated because the fellow eye can be involved within hours to days. In regard to systemic workup, it should be noted that patients with acute central artery obstruction have a high death rate from cardiac vascular disease.

If iris neovascularization develops, laser panretinal photocoagulation (PRP) should be considered to help prevent neovascular glaucoma. It causes resolution of the new iris vessels in approximately two thirds of treated cases.

ACUTE OPHTHALMIC ARTERY OBSTRUCTION (OCCLUSION)

Definition

This entity describes the acute blockage of the ophthalmic artery.

Epidemiology and Etiology

Acute ophthalmic artery obstruction occurs in approximately 1:100,000 ophthalmologic visits. The mean age of onset is in the sixties. No hereditary pattern is known.

Pathophysiology

Embolic

Trauma

Infectious (e.g., mucormycosis of the orbit)

Inflammatory (e.g., collagen vascular disease, giant cell arteritis)

Other (see causes of acute central retinal artery obstruction)

Clinical Features

Visual Acuity   Generally, there is a history of acute, unilateral, painless visual loss occurring over a period ranging from seconds. The visual acuity is no light perception in 90% of cases.

Pupillary Changes   An afferent pupillary defect is present.

Fundus Changes   Superficial retinal whitening in the posterior pole occurs, often more pronounced than with acute central retinal artery obstruction because the retinal pigment epithelium may be opacified as well with acute ophthalmic artery obstruction (Figure 4-13A). The presence of a cherry red spot in the foveola is variable; one third of patients have none, one third have a mild cherry red spot, and one third have a prominent cherry red spot.

The presence of retinal arterial emboli is variable. "Salt and pepper" retinal pigment

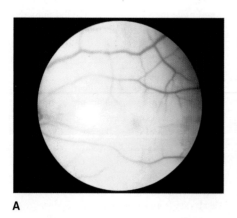 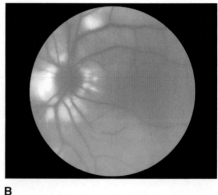

A   B

Figure 4-13   Acute ophthalmic artery obstruction   *A. Marked retinal whitening is present, and a cherry red spot is absent. The visual acuity was no light perception.* ***B.*** *Fluorescein angiogram corresponding to (A). At 116 seconds after injection, there is no dye within the retinal vessels and the majority of the choroid.*

CHAPTER 4.   RETINAL VASCULAR DISEASE

epithelial changes occur in the posterior pole and elsewhere within weeks after the acute obstruction. The pigment epithelial changes do not occur secondary to central retinal artery obstruction alone.

Differential Diagnosis

Refer to Table 4-1

Diagnostic Evaluation

Intravenous Fluorescein Angiography

Delay in choroidal filling—the choroid should be completely filled within 5 seconds after the first appearance of fluorescein dye within it (Figure 4-13B).
Delayed retinal arterial and venous filling.
Late focal or diffuse staining of the retinal pigment epithelium due to choroidal ischemia.

Electroretinography Decreased or absent a-wave (outer layer retinal ischemia) and b-wave (inner layer retinal ischemia) amplitudes.

Systemic Workup (This is similar to that of acute central retinal artery obstruction.)

Embolic—carotid and cardiac

Inflammatory—giant cell arteritis, Wegener's granulomatosis, polyarteritis nodosa, systemic lupus erythematosus, orbital mucormycosis, toxoplasmosis retinitis.
Coagulopathies—sickle cell disease, homocysteinuria, lupus anticoagulant syndrome, protein S deficiency, protein C deficiency, antithrombin III deficiency
Miscellaneous—fibromuscular hyperplasia, Sydenham's chorea, Fabry's disease, migraine, Lyme disease, hypotension

The most common etiology is as an iatrogenic sequela of retrobulbar injection.

Prognosis and Management

Although spontaneous reversal can rarely occur, the long-term vision in most cases is usually light perception to no light perception. There is no proven treatment to ameliorate the visual acuity. Despite the lack of an effective ocular treatment, a systemic workup should be undertaken.

The patient should be observed regularly for the first several months for the development of iris neovascularization. Laser PRP should be considered if iris neovascularization develops (the incidence of development of iris neovascularization is unknown).

TABLE 4-1   **DIFFERENTIAL DIAGNOSIS OF ACUTE OPHTHALMIC ARTERY OBSTRUCTION**

	Central Retinal Artery Obstruction	Ophthalmic Artery Obstruction
Vision	Finger counting — hand motions	No light perception
Fundus	Retinal opacification with cherry red spot	Marked opacification ± cherry red spot
Fluorescein angiography	Delayed retinal vascular filling	Delayed choroidal and retinal vascular filling
Electroretinography	Decreased b-wave	Decreased a- and b-waves

COMBINED CENTRAL RETINAL ARTERY AND VEIN OBSTRUCTION (OCCLUSION)

Definition

This entity describes the acute blockage of both the central retinal artery and the central retinal vein.

Epidemiology and Etiology

The prevalence is uncertain. No hereditary pattern is known.

Pathophysiology

The disease process is uncertain; blockage of both the central retinal artery and the central retinal vein has been shown in one case.

Clinical Signs

Visual Acuity Generally, there is a history of acute or subacute, unilateral, painless visual field loss occurring over a period ranging from seconds to days.

Pupillary Changes An afferent pupillary defect is typically present.

Fundus Changes (Figure 4-14)

   Superficial retinal whitening in the posterior pole
   Cherry red spot in the foveola
   Dilated, tortuous retinal veins
   Retinal hemorrhages
   Macular edema

Differential Diagnosis

   Inflammatory retinitis from cytomegalovirus
   Central retinal vein obstruction (no cherry red spot is present)

Diagnostic Evaluation

Intravenous Fluorescein Angiography
Reveals a delay in retinal arterial and venous filling in the area of obstruction versus the normal remaining fundus. Severe retinal capillary nonperfusion is often present.

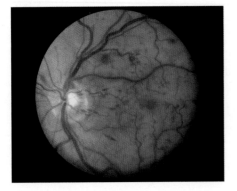

Figure 4-14   Combined central retinal artery and central retinal vein occlusion
The retinal veins are dilated and tortuous, retinal hemorrhages are present, and a cherry red spot due to superficial retinal opacification can be seen.

Systemic Workup   (This is similar to that of acute central retinal artery obstruction.)

Embolic—carotid and cardiac

Inflammatory—giant cell arteritis, Wegener's granulomatosis, polyarteritis nodosa, systemic lupus erythematosus, orbital mucormycosis, toxoplasmosis retinitis

Coagulopathies—sickle cell disease, homocysteinuria, lupus anticoagulant syndrome, protein S deficiency, protein C deficiency, antithrombin III deficiency

Miscellaneous—fibromuscular hyperplasia, Sydenham's chorea, Fabry's disease, migraine, Lyme disease, hypotension

The most common etiology is as a sequela of retrobulbar injection.

Prognosis and Management

Although there are exceptions, the vision most often remains in the counting fingers to light perception range. Approximately 80% of eyes will progress to iris neovascularization at a mean time of approximately 6 weeks after the obstruction.

There is no proven treatment to ameliorate the visual acuity. Despite the lack of an effective ocular treatment, a systemic workup should be undertaken. The patient should be followed regularly for the first several months for the development of iris neovascularization. Laser PRP should be considered if iris neovascularization develops. If the visual acuity is counting fingers or worse, PRP can be considered prior to the development of iris neovascularization.

OCULAR ISCHEMIC SYNDROME

Definition

Ocular ischemic syndrome describes ocular symptoms and signs attributable to marked carotid or ophthalmic artery obstruction. Alternative nomenclatures include venous stasis retinopathy, ischemic ocular inflammation, and ischemic oculopathy.

Epidemiology and Etiology

Approximately 2000 cases occur in the United States per year. The entity is unilateral in 80% of cases and bilateral in 20%. It occurs in approximately 5% of patients with carotid artery obstruction and is not usually seen in those under the age of 50 years. The mean age is 65 years. No hereditary pattern is known.

Pathophysiology

Disease involves blockage of the carotid or ophthalmic artery, or both. No flow disturbance occurs until there is 70% obstruction. With 90% obstruction, perfusion pressure in the central retinal artery decreases by 50%. Half of cases have a 100% ipsilateral common or internal carotid artery obstruction. Causes include:

Atherosclerosis (over 90% of cases)
Giant cell arteritis

Clinical Features

Symptoms and Signs

Vision—decreases over a period of weeks to months, although in 12% there is acute visual loss associated with a cherry red spot.
Periorbital pain—"ocular angina" is present in about 40% of cases and is described as a dull ache.
Prolonged visual recovery time after exposure to bright light.

Pupillary changes—an afferent pupillary defect is typically present.

Anterior Segment

Iris neovascularization (67%)
Anterior chamber cells (20%)

Posterior Segment

Narrowed retinal arteries in most cases
Dilated, but not tortuous, retinal veins (Figure 4-15A) in most cases
Microaneurysms (Figure 4-15C) in most cases (posterior pole or peripheral, or both)
Retinal dot and blot hemorrhages (80% of eyes)
Neovascularization of the optic disc and/or retina (35%)
Superficial retinal whitening in the posterior pole (12%)
Macular edema (Figure 4-15B) (11%)
Spontaneous retinal arterial pulsations (4%)

Associated Systemic Abnormalities

Systemic arterial hypertension (65%)
Cardiac disease (50%)
Diabetes mellitus (50%)
Previous stroke (20%)
Severe peripheral vascular disease (20%)

Differential Diagnosis

Central retinal vein obstruction typically has tortuous retinal veins, as well as more retinal hemorrhages and macular edema than the ocular ischemic syndrome. Light digital pressure on the lid, or minimal pressure with ophthalmodynamometry, will induce retinal arterial pulsations with the ocular ischemic syndrome, whereas substantial pressure is required with central retinal vein occlusion. Also consider:

Diabetic retinopathy
Radiation retinopathy

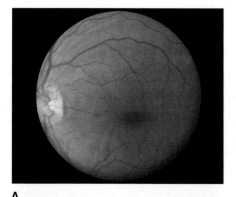

A

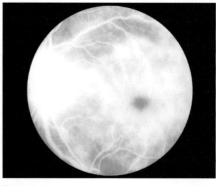

B

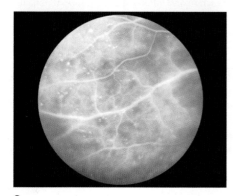

C

Figure 4-15   Ocular ischemic syndrome
A. The retinal veins are slightly dilated, but not tortuous, and the retinal arteries are narrowed. A few retinal hemorrhages are noted in the macula. B. Fluorescein angiogram corresponding to (A). Hyperfluorescence of the optic disc and macular edema are prominent. C. Fluorescein angiogram in an eye with ocular ischemic syndrome demonstrating pinpoint foci of hyperfluorescence due to microaneurysms in the midperipheral fundus.

Diagnostic Evaluation

Intravenous Fluorescein Angiography
Delay in choroidal filling (Figure 4-16) occurs in 60% of cases. Delayed retinal arterial and venous filling (see Figure 4-16) occurs in 95% of cases. Late retinal vascular staining, more pronounced of the retinal arteries (Figure 4-17), occurs in 85% of cases.

Electroretinography Decreased or absent a-wave (outer layer retinal ischemia) and b-wave (inner layer retinal ischemia) amplitudes are seen.

Systemic Workup Carotid noninvasive studies have approximately 90% chance of detecting carotid stenosis of 50% or more. Carotid arteriography or magnetic resonance angiography (MRA) is performed if carotid noninvasive studies are ambiguous or if carotid artery surgery is being considered.

Prognosis

Ocular—75% of eyes will progress to counting fingers of worse vision within 1 year after diagnosis.

Systemic—there is a 40% 5-year mortality, with cardiac disease as the most common cause of death.

Management

Laser PRP is performed if there is iris neovascularization and the anterior chamber angle is open. PRP induces regression of iris new vessels in 36% of cases. The patient should be evaluated for possible carotid endarterectomy. In surgical candidates, one third demonstrate improved vision, one third demonstrate stabilized vision, and one third progress to lose vision despite endarterectomy surgery.

If the carotid artery is 100% obstructed, endarterectomy is not of benefit; neither is extracranial to intracranial (e.g., superficial temporal to middle cerebral) bypass. Remember not to ignore the cardiac status, because cardiac disease is the leading cause of death.

Endarterectomy is indicated for symptomatic patients (those with amaurosis fugax, transient ischemic attack, or nondisabling stroke), and those with 70% to 99% ipsilateral carotid stenosis (Table 4-2). Antiplatelet therapy is indicated for those who are symptomatic and have less than 70% stenosis.

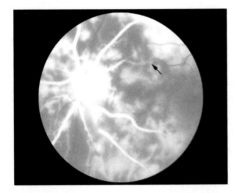

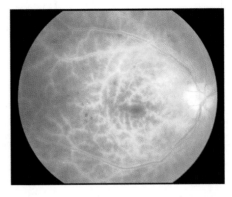

Figure 4-16 Ocular ischemic syndrome
Fluorescein angiogram revealing delayed retinal arterial and choroidal vascular filling in an ocular ischemic syndrome eye. Note the abnormal leading edge of fluorescein dye in the retinal arteriole (arrow).

Figure 4-17 Ocular ischemic syndrome
Late-phase fluorescein angiogram demonstrating retinal vascular staining in an ocular ischemic syndrome eye.

TABLE 4-2 **OUTCOMES AFTER TREATMENT OF SYMPTOMATIC PATIENTS WITH HIGH-GRADE CAROTID ARTERY STENOSIS[a]**

	Endarterectomy	Antiplatelet Agent
Perioperative mortality	2%	1%
Severe stroke by 2 years	9%	26%

[a]North American Symptomatic Carotid Endarterectomy Trial (NASCET) data.

BRANCH RETINAL VEIN OBSTRUCTION (OCCLUSION)

Definition

This entity describes the acute blockage of blood flow within a branch retinal vein.

Epidemiology and Etiology

Branch retinal vein obstruction typically occurs in patients aged 65 years and older but can be seen at any age. The Beaver Dam Eye Study noted a prevalence of 0.6% and a 5-year incidence of 0.6% as well. No hereditary pattern is known.

Pathophysiology

Branch retinal vein occlusion typically occurs at a retinal arteriovenous crossing. Impingement of the branch retinal artery on the branch retinal vein is believed to cause turbulent flow, leading to endothelial cell damage and predisposing to thrombus formation within the branch retinal vein.

When the branch retinal vein occlusion does not occur at an arteriovenous crossing, an inflammatory cause, such as sarcoidosis, should be considered.

Clinical Signs

Visual Acuity   Generally, there is a history of unilateral, painless visual loss occurring over a period of days.

Pupillary Changes   An afferent pupillary defect may be present, depending on the size of the venous occlusion and the degree of retinal ischemia.

Anterior Segment Changes   Iris neovascularization has been observed to develop in 5% to 10% of hemispheric retinal vein occlusions and 1% to 2% of branch retinal vein obstructions.

Posterior Segment Changes   Retinal venous engorgement and tortuosity, as well as retinal hemorrhages and edema, are typically present within the distribution of the occluded vessel (Figure 4-18A). Macular branch (twig) vein occlusions may be clinically subtle with minimal hemorrhage, telangiectasia, or macular edema.

Neovascularization of the optic disc or retina, or both, can develop months to years after the occlusion. Vitreous traction on retinal or optic disc neovascularization may lead to vitreous hemorrhage with or without traction retinal detachment.

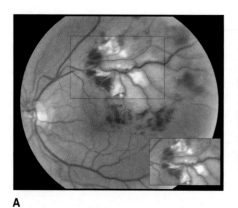
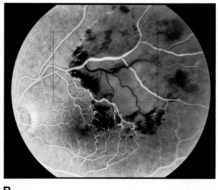

A　　　　　　　　　　　　　　　　　**B**

Figure 4-18　Branch retinal vein occlusion　*A. Retinal hemorrhages and cotton-wool spots are present in the distribution of the occluded vessel (inset).* ***B.*** *Fluorescein angiogram corresponding to (**A**). Retinal capillary nonperfusion is present in the distribution of the occluded vessel.*

　　　　　　　　　　　　　　　　　CHAPTER 4.   RETINAL VASCULAR DISEASE

Differential Diagnosis

Retinal cavernous hemangioma can occasionally mimic the appearance of a branch retinal vein occlusion.

Diagnostic Evaluation

Intravenous Fluorescein Angiography
Reveals a delay in retinal arterial and venous filling in the distribution of the obstructed vessel. Retinal capillary nonperfusion may be present (Figure 4-18B).

Systemic Workup   Includes an evaluation for systemic arterial hypertension and increased body mass. A history of glaucoma has also been associated with branch retinal vein occlusion.

Prognosis and Management

The mean resultant visual acuity in eyes with untreated branch retinal vein occlusion is 20/70. In eyes that are candidates for grid laser photocoagulation for macular edema, the mean visual result is 20/40 to 20/50.

According to the Branch Vein Occlusion Study, laser grid photocoagulation for visual loss due to macular edema can be considered for eyes with branch retinal occlusion that meet the following criteria:

Visual acuity of 20/40 to 20/200
Intact perifoveolar capillaries with fluorescein angiography
Resolution of the majority of intraretinal blood

If posterior segment neovascularization develops, sector laser PRP in the distribution of the obstructed branch retinal vein should be considered. This therapy reduces the incidence of subsequent vitreous hemorrhage from approximately 60% to 30%.

If iris neovascularization develops, sector laser PRP should be considered to help prevent neovascular glaucoma.

CENTRAL RETINAL VEIN OBSTRUCTION (OCCLUSION)

Definition

This entity describes blockage of blood flow within the central retinal vein.

Epidemiology and Etiology

Central retinal vein obstruction typically occurs in patients aged 65 years and older but can be seen at any age. In the Beaver Dam Eye study, the prevalence was 0.1% and the 5-year incidence was 0.2%. Bilaterality eventually occurs in approximately 10% of cases, more commonly in those with underlying systemic abnormalities. No hereditary pattern is known.

Pathophysiology

Green and associates (*Trans Am Ophthalmol Soc,* 1981; 79:371–422) demonstrated an intravenous thrombus at or near the lamina cribrosa in 29 of 29 eyes with central retinal vein obstruction studied histopathologically. Impingement of the central retinal artery on the central retinal vein is believed to cause turbulence and subsequent endothelial damage, which predisposes to thrombus formation.

Increased intraocular pressure may also predispose to central retinal vein obstruction by theoretically bowing the lamina cribrosa posteriorly, leading to turbulence, endothelial damage, and thrombus formation.

Clinical Signs

Visual Acuity   Generally, there is a history of unilateral, painless visual loss occurring over hours to days or weeks. Nonischemic central retinal vein occlusions (Figure 4-19) typically are associated with vision of 20/200

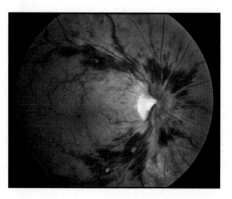

Figure 4-19   Nonischemic central retinal vein occlusion   *Note the retinal hemorrhages in all four quadrants around the optic disc. The visual acuity in the eye was 20/50.*

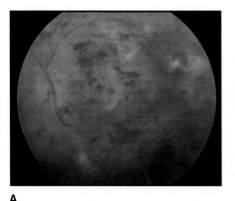 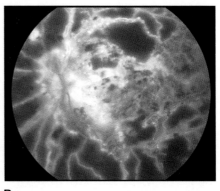

A   **B**

Figure 4-20   Ischemic central retinal occlusion *A. Retinal hemorrhage, diffuse retinal edema, and numerous cotton-wool spots are present. The visual acuity was hand motions.* ***B.*** *Fluorescein angiogram corresponding to (**A**). Areas of marked retinal capillary nonperfusion and macular edema are present. Some of the areas of hypofluorescence correspond to retinal hemorrhages. (continued)*

or better, whereas ischemic central retinal vein obstructions (Figure 4-20A–E) are associated with vision of counting fingers or worse.

Approximately 20% of eyes with nonischemic central retinal vein occlusion will eventually progress to the ischemic variant.

Pupillary Changes An afferent pupillary defect may be present, increasing in severity as the visual acuity decreases and the degree of ischemia increases.

Anterior Segment Changes Iris neovascularization (rubeosis iridis) develops in approxi-

mately 20% of cases at a mean time of 3 to 5 months after the obstruction.

Posterior Segment Changes

Dilated, tortuous retinal veins

Retinal hemorrhages, most pronounced in the posterior pole

Retinal edema, most pronounced in the macula

Neovascularization of the optic disc or retina, or both, or optic disc collaterals (Figure 4-20F); may develop months after the obstruction

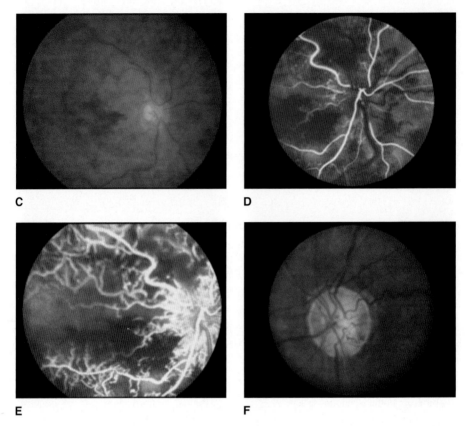

C

D

E

F

Figure 4-20 (cont.) **Ischemic central retinal occlusion** *C. Retinal hemorrhage, retinal venous tortuosity, diffuse macular edema, and markedly narrowed retinal arterioles are present. D. Fluorescein angiogram corresponding to (C). Delayed retinal venous filling and retinal telangiectasia are noted. There is marked hypofluorescence from retinal ischemia and blockage from retinal hemorrhages. E. Fluorescein angiogram corresponding to (C). There is widespread macular ischemia. F. Optic disc collaterals shunting retinal venous blood to the choroidal circulation may be noted on the optic disc.*

Differential Diagnosis

Differential diagnosis includes ocular ischemic syndrome (Table 4-3). Diabetic retinopathy can also mimic central retinal vein obstruction, but the former is typically bilateral, has prominent hard exudates (rare in central retinal vein obstruction) and many more microaneurysms than with central retinal vein obstruction.

Diagnostic Evaluation

Intravenous Fluorescein Angiography
Reveals delay in retinal venous filling and intraretinal leakage of dye, most prominent in the macula, as the study progresses. Increasing areas of retinal capillary nonperfusion can be seen in more ischemic cases. When the retinal capillary nonperfusion (in seven fundus photographic

TABLE 4-3 DIFFERENTIAL DIAGNOSIS OF CENTRAL RETINAL VEIN OBSTRUCTION

	Central Retinal Vein Obstruction	Ocular Ischemic Syndrome
Vision	20/20—hand motions	20/20—no light perception
Iris neovascularization	20%	67%
Retinal hemorrhages	Mild to severe	Mild
Retinal venous tortuosity	Usually present	Absent
Macular edema	Mild to severe	Mild
Fluorescein angiography		
Choroidal filling	Normal	Delayed
Retinal AV transit	Delayed	Delayed
Late arterial staining	Absent	Present

AV = arteriovenous.

fields) exceeds 75 disc areas, the incidence of development of iris neovascularization rises to more than 50%.

Electroretinography Normal a-wave amplitude, but diminished b-wave amplitude, occurs as ischemia increases.

Systemic Workup

Systemic arterial hypertension

Diabetes mellitus

Hyperviscosity syndromes (e.g., polycythemia vera, Waldenstrom's macroglobulinemia, plasma cell dyscrasias such as multiple myeloma)

Hyperlipidemias

Inflammatory or infectious (e.g., sarcoidosis, systemic lupus erythematosus, syphilis)

Hypercoagulability states (e.g., lupus anticoagulant syndrome, protein S deficiency, protein C deficiency, antithrombin III deficiency, hyperhomocysteinemia)

Prognosis and Management

The visual prognosis is largely dependent on the presenting visual acuity at the time of initial diagnosis (Table 4-4). There is no consistently proven treatment to ameliorate the visual acuity. Treatment with systemic fibrinolytic agents, laser-induced retinochoroidal anastomosis, and macular grid laser photocoagulation has been attempted with limited success.

According to the guidelines of the Central Retinal Vein Occlusion Study, if any anterior chamber angle neovascularization or 2 clock hours or more of iris neovascularization develops, laser PRP should be considered to help prevent neovascular glaucoma.

TABLE 4-4 PROGNOSIS FOR CENTRAL RETINAL VEIN OCCLUSION

Initial Visual Acuity	Final Visual Acuity
≥ 20/40	65% with ≥ 20/40
20/50–20/200	19% > 20/50; 44% 20/50–20/200; 37% < 20/200
< 20/200	80% with < 20/200

RETINAL ARTERIAL MACROANEURYSM

Definition

First described in 1973, this abnormality is characterized by the presence of vascular dilation or outpouching of a retinal artery or arteriole.

Epidemiology

Retinal arterial macroaneurysms occur as isolated phenomena in two thirds of cases. About one third of cases are seen in conjunction in with retinal venous obstructions. Ten percent of cases are bilateral.

Pathophysiology

The aneurysms are believed to be clinically similar in size (300 μm) to the intracerebral variant, although no association with intracerebral aneurysms has been convincingly demonstrated. They can occur as saccular dilations within the vessel, or as outpouchings from the vessel. About three quarters of cases are associated with systemic arterial hypertension.

Clinical Signs

The entity is typically unilateral and isolated. Pulsations of the macroaneurysm are occasionally seen. The two most common variants of presentation are:

1. *Acute hemorrhage*—may develop in the subretinal space, retinal or preretinal region if the macroaneurysms ruptures. A multilevel hemorrhage should arouse suspicion of the presence of a macroaneurysm. A white or yellow spot (the aneurysm) is often present centrally within the hemorrhage (Figure 4-21). Recurrent bleeding is extremely unusual.
2. *Retinal edema*—may be the presenting sign when chronic leakage of plasma encroaches upon the fovea. In this instance, lipid exudation is also often present.

In approximately 4% of cases, a retinal arterial obstruction distal to the macroaneurysm is seen at the time of presentation.

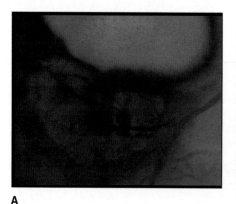 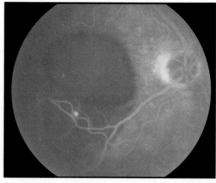

A   B

Figure 4-21   Retinal arterial macroaneurysm associated with yellowed blood
A. The blood superiorly is superficial to the retinal vessels (preretinal), *whereas inferiorly it is located in the subretinal space. The yellow macroaneurysm* (arrow) *is present along the course of the retinal artery. B. Fluorescein angiogram corresponding to* (A). *The aneurysm is hyperfluorescent and located along the inferotemporal retinal artery.*

CHAPTER 4.   RETINAL VASCULAR DISEASE

Differential Diagnosis

The abnormality is relatively unique in appearance. Aneurysmal abnormalities associated with Coats' disease can occasionally cause bleeding seen with retinal arterial macroaneurysms, but with Coats' disease there are typically multiple aneurysmal arterial or venous dilations, or both.

The presence of multiple, bilateral arterial aneurysmal abnormalities occurring principally at arterial bifurcations has been described with the disorder, termed idiopathic retinal vasculitis, aneurysms, and neuroretinitis (IRVAN).

Diagnostic Evaluation

Intravenous fluorescein angiography reveals hyperfluorescence corresponding to the macroaneurysm (Figure 4-21B). Vascular telangiectasias surrounding the aneurysmal abnormality may be present.

Prognosis and Management

The visual prognosis depends on whether bleeding involves the central macular region. In such instances, vision can be reduced to counting fingers or worse. Spontaneous improvement can occur, particularly when the blood is located superficially within the retina. Involvement of the macula by edema can lead to visual loss, typically ranging from 20/25 to 20/200.

The bleeding associated with macroaneurysms is not typically treated. It is usually a one-time event, and visual improvement can occur when the hemorrhage is located primarily within the superficial layers of the retina.

Although there are no randomized clinical studies addressing the issue, most retinal experts recommend treating the macroaneurysms when there is involvement of the central fovea by retinal edema or hard exudation, or both. Treatment is given using 200- to 500-μm spot size, light argon laser burns to the aneurysm and the retina surrounding the abnormality. In approximately 16% of cases, treatment leads to a retinal arterial obstruction distal to the aneurysm. Thus, treatment of aneurysms that could lead to an arterial obstruction involving the central macula should be undertaken with caution.

PARAFOVEAL TELANGIECTASIS

Definition

Parafoveal (juxtafoveal) telangiectasis is a retinal vascular entity characterized by the presence of incompetent retinal capillaries in the foveal region of one or both eyes.

Epidemiology and Etiology

Group 1 parafoveal telangiectasis has been associated with an abnormal glucose tolerance in more than 30% of cases. Group 2 parafoveal telangiectasis has been associated with an abnormal glucose tolerance test in more than 60% of cases. The incidence of parafoveal telangiectasis is uncertain. There is no known hereditary pattern.

Pathophysiology

Histopathology has shown thickening of the walls of the retinal capillaries by a deposition of basement membrane. The changes are similar to those seen with diabetic retinopathy.

Clinical Signs

The entity is stratified into three variants:

Group 1—unilateral parafoveal telangiectasis
Group 2—bilateral parafoveal telangiectasis
Group 3—bilateral occlusive parafoveolar telangiectasis alone or associated with central nervous system occlusive vasculitis

There is typically a blunted foveolar reflex with localized retinal thickening most pronounced in the temporal fovea. A grayish macular reflex may be observed clinically and highlighted with red-free photography. Retinal pigment epithelial hyperplasia, most prominent in the temporal fovea, can been seen in the later stages, as can right-angle venules diving into the outer retina. Yellow intraretinal crystals in the fovea are also seen in some cases (Figure 4-22A). Despite the retinal thickening, the retinal cystoid changes often seen with diabetic retinopathy or retinal vein obstruction are not usually present with parafoveal telangiectasis.

In approximately 5% of patients, choroidal neovascularization can develop in the region of the telangiectatic retinal vessels.

Differential Diagnosis

Diabetic retinopathy
Radiation retinopathy
Carotid obstructive disease (ocular ischemic syndrome)
Twig retinal vein obstruction
Coats' disease
Macular edema associated with the Irvine-Gass syndrome
Macular edema associated with uveitis

The appearance of temporal foveal leakage with fluorescein angiography is very helpful for making the diagnosis of parafoveal telangiectasis. In contrast to the Irvine-Gass syndrome (macular edema after cataract surgery) or uveitis associated with macular edema, the optic disc is not usually hyperfluorescent in eyes with parafoveal telangiectasis.

Diagnostic Evaluation

The ophthalmoscopic diagnosis is often difficult. Intravenous fluorescein angiography is often required to make the diagnosis. There is characteristic intraretinal leakage of dye located primarily in the temporal macula (Figure 4-22B,C). In the group 3 variant, areas of retinal capillary dropout can be seen in the foveal region.

Prognosis and Management

When patients first present, the visual acuity is often only mildly decreased to the 20/20 to 20/30 range. Over the years, the vision can decrease dramatically to legal blindness. When abrupt loss of vision is present, the possibility of an associated choroidal neovascular membrane should be considered.

Laser photocoagulation has not been shown to be of benefit for the treatment of parafoveal telangiectasis. Laser therapy may be of benefit in treating the choroidal neovascularization associated with parafoveal telangiectasis. Patients should be made aware of the strong association between an abnormal glucose tolerance test and parafoveal telangiectasis, especially the group 2 variant.

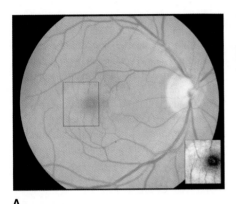

A

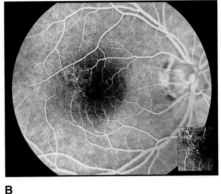

B

Figure 4-22 Group 2 parafoveal telangiectasis *A. The temporal foveal retina is thickened, and crystalline deposits are present in this area as well. The visual acuity in the eye was 20/100. Inset highlights telangiectatic changes.* ***B.*** *Early-phase fluorescein angiogram corresponding to (**A**). Telangiectatic retinal vascular changes are present surrounding the foveal avascular zone.* ***C.*** *Late-phase fluorescein angiogram corresponding to (**A**). Intraretinal leakage of dye is present in the vicinity of the telangiectatic changes in the temporal fovea.*

C

SICKLE CELL RETINOPATHY

Definition

This entity describes the fundus changes associated with sickle cell hemoglobinopathies.

Epidemiology

Approximately 10% of the U.S. population has any form of sickle hemoglobin; 0.4% have hemoglobin SS, 0.2% have hemoglobin SC, and 0.03% have sickle cell thalassemia (SThal).

Proliferative sickle retinopathy has been noted to occur in Jamaican individuals with sickle hemoglobinopathy in the following percentages: SS, 3%; SC, 33%; and SThal, 14%.

Pathophysiology

Sickled red blood cells cause obstruction within the retinal vasculature. Multiple hemoglobin variants have been described, along with their genetic changes. Although SS disease is associated with more severe systemic disease, SC disease causes more advanced ocular disease.

Clinical Signs

Nonproliferative Manifestations

Salmon patch hemorrhage—an oval-shaped area of intraretinal or preretinal blood believed to occur secondary to an obstructed retinal arteriole, which subsequently ruptures.

Iridescent spot—a small retinoschisis cavity within the superficial retina that can occur as a salmon patch resolves. It is filled with hemosiderin-laden macrophages.

Black sunburst lesion (Figure 4-23)—an oval or round collection of retinal pigment epithelial cells that are believed to develop from a salmon patch hemorrhage that has dissected into the subretinal space or from a focal choroidal occlusion.

Proliferative Changes

Five stages have been described:

Stage I—peripheral retinal arteriolar occlusions
Stage II—peripheral retinal arteriovenous anastomoses
Stage III—peripheral retinal neovascularization ("sea fans") (Figure 4-24A)
Stage IV—vitreous hemorrhage
Stage V—rhegmatogenous or traction retinal detachment, or both

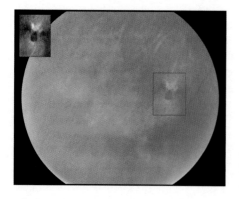

Figure 4-23   Sickle cell retinopathy, "black sunburst lesion"   *Small, black sunburst lesion* (inset) *in an eye with sickle cell retinopathy. There is a sclerotic retinal vessel leading to ischemic peripheral retina inferiorly.*

CHAPTER 4.   RETINAL VASCULAR DISEASE

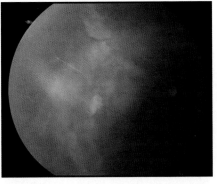

A

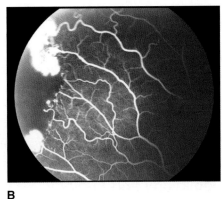

B

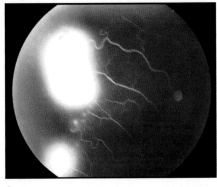

C

Figure 4-24   Stage 3 proliferative sickle cell retinopathy *A. Orange "sea fans," or areas of peripheral retinal neovascularization, are present at the juncture of perfused and ischemic peripheral retina. **B.** Fluorescein angiogram corresponding to (**A**) at 29 seconds after injection. The sea fans are hyperfluorescent, and retinal capillary nonperfusion is visible adjacent to them on the left side of the photo. **C.** Late-phase fluorescein angiogram showing marked leakage of fluorescein dye into the vitreous from the retinal sea fan neovascularization.*

Differential Diagnosis

Eales' disease
Proliferative diabetic retinopathy
Radiation retinopathy
Retinal vein occlusion
Sarcoidosis

Diagnostic Evaluation

A history of sickle cell disease may be elicited, and thus a sickle cell prep or hemoglobin electrophoresis should be considered when characteristic findings are noted.

The disease is diagnosed by its clinical appearance. Intravenous fluorescein angiography reveals retinal capillary nonperfusion adjacent and peripheral to areas of peripheral retinal neovascularization (Figure 4-24A–C).

Prognosis and Management

The visual prognosis is often relatively good unless the sequelae of proliferative sickle disease (vitreous hemorrhage or retinal detachment, or both) develop.

Treatment is not indicated for the nonproliferative changes of sickling hemoglobinopathies. When peripheral retinal neovascularization is present, full scatter laser photocoagulation to the retina peripheral to the neovascularization has been shown to reduce the incidence of subsequent vitreous hemorrhage. Many have advocated treating the peripheral retina for 360 degrees.

Para plana vitrectomy can be of benefit for chronic vitreous hemorrhage. Vitrectomy, with or without scleral buckling, may be of benefit for the repair of retinal detachment.

RADIATION RETINOPATHY

Definition

This entity describes the damage induced to the retina or optic nerve, or both, by external beam irradiation (teletherapy) or by localized irradiation (brachytherapy). The optic nerve changes are referred to as radiation optic neuropathy.

Epidemiology and Etiology

Damage from external beam irradiation often occurs from irradiation to structures adjacent to the eyes (brain, oropharynx, etc.). Typically, a minimum dose of 1500 cGy (centigray) of external beam irradiation is required to induce retinopathy. The mean dose is about 5000 cGy. At a dose of 7000 to 8000 cGy, 85% of eyes will develop radiation retinopathy. Fraction sizes of more than 200 per day appear to amplify the chances of radiation damage. For ^{60}Co brachytherapy, a minimum of 20,000 cGy to the tumor base is necessary to induce radiation changes, with the average dose over 30,000 cGy.

Pathophysiology

Radiation retinopathy and optic neuropathy are caused primarily by damage to the vasculature of the respective structures.

Clinical Signs

Radiation changes usually occur at a mean time of 12 to 18 months after the termination of radiation, with a range from 1 month to 7 years. The condition can be unilateral or bilateral, depending on the fields included in the irradiation.

Visual acuity is variable, depending on the degree of damage to the retinal or optic nerve vasculature.

The retinal changes (Figure 4-25A–C) are characterized by the presence of cotton-wool spots, retinal hemorrhages, and hard exudation. Neovascularization of the optic disc or retina, or both, can develop as well. Optic nerve changes are characterized by disc edema, at times in conjunction with peripapillary subretinal fluid and lipid exudation (Figure 4-26). Retinopathy and optic neuropathy can occur concomitantly or separately.

The fundus findings with brachytherapy are similar to those with teletherapy (Figure 4-27), although hard exudation tends to be a more prominent feature with brachytherapy (Figure 4-28).

Differential Diagnosis

Radiation retinopathy can closely mimic diabetic retinopathy. There are usually more microaneurysms present with diabetic retinopathy than with radiation retinopathy. Key to the diagnosis of radiation is the elicitation of a history of radiation to or around the eyes.

Diagnostic Evaluation

Intravenous fluorescein angiography reveals retinal capillary dropout, retinal vascular telangiectases, and late leakage of dye from the damaged vessels.

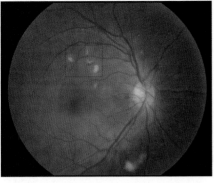

A

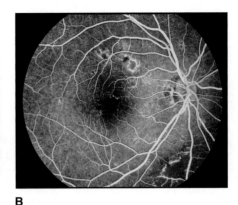

B

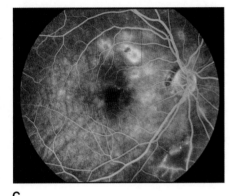

C

Figure 4-25   Radiation retinopathy after teletherapy   *A. Cotton-wool spots and small retinal hemorrhage are present in the posterior pole. **B.** Fluorescein angiogram corresponding to (A) at 25 seconds after injection. The cotton-wool spots are hypofluorescent. Note the radiation-induced capillary telangiectasia at the fovea and below the inferior retinal vascular arcade where capillary nonperfusion is noted. **C.** Fluorescein angiogram corresponding to (A) at 375 seconds after injections. The cotton-wool spots are now more hyperfluorescent due to leakage of dye from the retina at their border.*

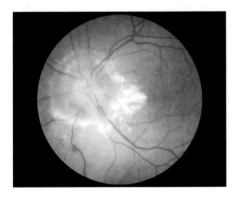

Figure 4-26   Radiation optic neuropathy after teletherapy   *The optic disc is swollen and surrounded by peripapillary lipid exudates and subretinal fluid.*

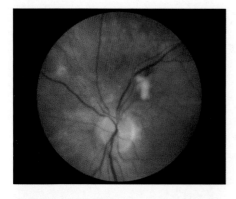

Figure 4-27 Radiation retinopathy following brachytherapy for a choroidal melanoma *Cotton-wool spots are present in the peripapillary region.*

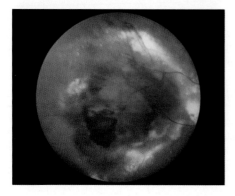

Figure 4-28 Radiation retinopathy surrounding a choroidal melanoma treated with brachytherapy *Marked lipid exudation is present at the necrotic tumor base.*

Prognosis and Management

The visual prognosis depends on the dose of radiation received. The presence of chemotherapy, systemic arterial hypertension, diabetic retinopathy, and other diseases that can damage the retinal vasculature appear to be additive to the radiation damage.

With brachytherapy for choroidal melanoma, about two thirds of eyes have 20/200 vision or better at 2 to 3 years after treatment.

Approximately 25% untreated eyes with radiation retinopathy from external beam irradi-

ation progress to develop iris neovascularization of the iris and neovascular glaucoma.

Macular edema can be treated with focal laser therapy in a fashion similar to the treatment of clinically significant macular edema in the Early Treatment Diabetic Retinopathy Study. Laser PRP is indicated when neovascularization of the iris or posterior segment neovascularization develops.

There is no known effective treatment for radiation optic neuropathy, but spontaneous improvement of vision occurs in about 20% of cases.

LIPEMIA RETINALIS

Definition

Lipemia retinalis refers to salmon-colored retinal arteries and retinal veins due to elevated lipids, most commonly hypertriglyceridemia.

Pathophysiology

Elevated serum lipid levels may cause retinal vascular obstruction. The lipid abnormalities are typically heritable lipid metabolic abnormalities.

Clinical Signs

Pale conjunctiva may result from lipemic conjunctival blood vessels. Fundus examination reveals salmon-colored retinal arteries and veins without skip areas (Figure 4-29A,B).

Differential Diagnosis

Retinal vascular whitening can be observed in prior retinal vascular occlusion or in retinal vasculitidies. These are typically confined to the retinal arterial or venous systems and typically have skip segments where the retinal vasculature is unaffected. Lipemia retinalis shows diffuse retinal arterial and venous involvement.

Diagnostic Evaluation

Fundus biomicroscopic examination reveals the characteristic retinal appearance described earlier and usually suffices to prompt systemic lipid evaluation. Fluorescein angiography may be obtained to evaluate retinal perfusion; areas of retinal telangiectasia may be observed. Family members should be evaluated, and systemic evaluation is indicated because of potential problems such as pancreatitis.

Prognosis and Management

The visual prognosis can be good for patients who do not develop retinal vascular occlusive disease. Treatment is directed toward decreasing the causative lipemic factor.

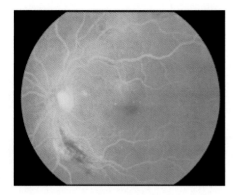

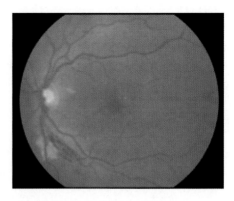

Figure 4-29A   Lipemia retinalis *A patient with markedly elevated triglyceride lipid levels who presented with a branch retinal vein occlusion and lipemic yellow retinal vessels and microaneurysms.*

Figure 4-29B   Lipemia retinalis, posttreatment *After treatment with oral lipid-lowering agents, the retinal vasculature assumes normal coloring.*

Chapter 5

CHORIORETINAL INFLAMMATORY DISEASES

Magdalena F. Shuler, MD

Carl D. Regillo, MD

INFECTIOUS CAUSES

Endophthalmitis

ACUTE POSTOPERATIVE ENDOPHTHALMITIS

Definition   Acute postoperative endophthalmitis describes an intraocular infection with vitreous involvement after recent ocular surgery (within 6 weeks).

Epidemiology and Etiology

CAUSES   Infection can occur after any intraocular surgery. Clinical course depends on the infectious cause. Infectious organisms include *Staphylococcus epidermidis,* 68%; other grampositive organisms such as *Staphylococcus aureus* and *Streptococcus* species, 22%; gramnegative species, 6%.

INCIDENCE   Between 0.07% and 0.12% after cataract surgery, 0.11% after penetrating keratoplasty, 0.05% after vitrectomy.

History   Patients present with an abrupt onset of floaters, decreased vision, and pain.

Important Clinical Signs   Hypopyon with vitritis after recent surgery (Figure 5-1).

Associated Clinical Signs   Conjunctival injection and chemosis. Patients may sometimes have corneal stromal infiltrate or ulceration at wound site or scleral thinning at wound site.

Differential Diagnosis

Postoperative inflammation

Diagnostic Evaluation   Diagnosis is based on clinical examination. Ultrasonography shows vitritis and often some degree of scleralchoroidal thickening. Undiluted vitreous sample is obtained for cultures and sensitivities.

Prognosis and Management   Prognosis depends mainly on causative bacteria. *Staphylococcus epidermidis* is the most commonly isolated bacteria and carries the most favorable

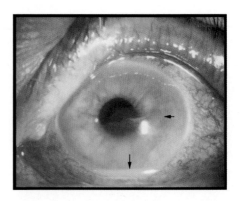

Figure 5-1   Endophthalmitis   *Patient with conjunctival injection and edema, corneal edema, fibrinous anterior chamber reaction* (short arrow), *and hypopyon* (long arrow).

TABLE 5-1 ENDOPHTHALMITIS VITRECTOMY STUDY

Presenting Vision		Visual Outcomes			Recommended Treatment
		20/40 or better	20/100 or better	Less than 5/100	
HM or better	TAP	62%	84%	3%	TAP
	PPV	66%	86%	5%	
LP	TAP	11%	30%	47%	PPV
	PPV	33%	56%	20%	

HM = hand motions vision at 2 feet, LP = light perception, PPV = pars plana vitrectomy and intravitreal injection of antibiotics, TAP = vitreous tap and intravitreal injection of antibiotics.

prognosis, with 61.5% of cases recovering better than 20/40 vision with treatment. *Staphylococcus aureus*, *Streptococcus* species, and gram-negative bacteria are less commonly isolated and carry a poor visual prognosis.

The need for vitrectomy is based on vision at presentation (Table 5-1). *Intravitreal antibiotics:* vancomycin (1 mg/0.1 mL) and amikacin (400 μg/0.1 mL), or ceftazidime (2.25 mg/0.1 mL). *Topical antibiotics:* fortified vancomycin (25 mg/mL), cefazolin (50 mg/mL), amikacin (20 mg/mL), tobramycin (15 mg/mL), or ciprofloxacin. Topical steroids and intravitreal steroids (dexamethasone 400 μg/0.1 mL) can be considered.

LATE-ONSET ENDOPHTHALMITIS

Definition This entity describes intraocular infection involving the vitreous cavity after previous ocular surgery (more than 6 weeks).

Epidemiology and Etiology

CAUSES The usual causative organism is *Propionibacterium acnes,* but infection may also be caused by *Staphylococcus epidermidis* or fungi.

PRESENTATION May occur up to 2 or more years after surgery.

History Patients have variably decreased vision with photophobia, and a gradual onset of symptoms. Infection may be painless.

Important Clinical Signs Vitritis, with or without hypopyon, more than 4 to 6 weeks after surgery; anterior chamber keratic precipitates; white plaque on intraocular lens or posterior lens capsule.

Associated Clinical Signs Conjunctival injection.

Differential Diagnosis

Postoperative inflammation
Rebound inflammation after discontinuing steroids

Diagnostic Evaluation Diagnosis is based on clinical examination, and ultrasonography showing vitritis and variable scleral-choroidal thickening.

Prognosis and Management Intravitreal tap and injection of vancomycin (or clindamycin, 1 mg/0.1 mL) may not be curative. Patients may require vitrectomy with capsulotomy or, sometimes, explantation of the intraocular lens and entire lens capsule.

ENDOPHTHALMITIS VITRECTOMY STUDY (EVS)

The goal of this nationwide, collaborative study was to determine the management of patients presenting with endophthalmitis within 6 weeks of cataract surgery with lens implantation or secondary lens implantation. Visual outcomes were determined for vitreous tap and intravitreal antibiotics versus vitrectomy and intravitreal antibiotics. Treatment recommendations were made based on presenting vision (see Table 5-1).

BLEB-ASSOCIATED ENDOPHTHALMITIS

Definition This term refers to intraocular infection involving the vitreous cavity anytime after glaucoma filtering surgery.

Epidemiology and Etiology

CAUSES *Streptococcus* species, *Haemophilus influenzae, Moraxella* species.

INCIDENCE Ranges from 0.2% to 9.60%. There is a greater risk with thin-walled blebs (postmitomycin) and inferior placement.

History Patients present with decreased vision accompanied by pain, conjunctival injection, and sometimes discharge.

Important Clinical Signs Opaque (infected) bleb; hypopyon with vitritis after glaucoma surgery.

Associated Clinical Signs Conjunctival injection and chemosis; purulent conjunctival discharge.

Differential Diagnosis

Postoperative inflammation
"Blebitis" (infection limited to the bleb site and anterior chamber)

Diagnostic Evaluation Diagnosis is based on clinical examination. Ultrasonography shows vitritis and variable scleral-choroidal thickening.

Prognosis and Management Prognosis is usually poor with severe vision loss. Treatment consists of intravitreal tap or vitrectomy and intravitreal injection of antibiotics (vancomycin and amikacin or ceftazidime). May consider following EVS criteria for vitrectomy.

TRAUMATIC ENDOPHTHALMITIS

Definition This term describes inflammation of the vitreous cavity after penetrating trauma.

Epidemiology and Etiology

CAUSES *Staphylococcus epidermidis, Bacillus* species; *Bacillus cereus* may cause a fulminate infection.

INCIDENCE Between 2.4% and 8% with penetrating trauma; 30% with retained intraocular foreign bodies.

History Patients present with decreasing vision and increasing pain.

Important Clinical Signs Hypopyon with increasing vitritis after penetrating trauma.

Associated Clinical Signs Conjunctival injection and chemosis.

Differential Diagnosis

Postoperative or traumatic inflammation
Sympathetic ophthalmia

Diagnostic Evaluation Diagnosis is based on clinical examination. Ultrasonography shows vitritis and variable scleral-choroidal thickening.

Prognosis and Management Prognosis is variable, usually poor for *Bacillus* species or *Streptococcus* species. Treatment involves intravitreal tap and injection of antibiotics (vancomycin and amikacin or ceftazidime). May consider following EVS criteria to determine need for vitrectomy.

Ocular Toxoplasmosis

Definition Ocular toxoplasmosis describes a focal area of chorioretinitis, which shows full-thickness inflammation and results in a pigmented scar. If the presentation is due to reactivation, an acute inflammatory lesion is adjacent to a chorioretinal scar.

Epidemiology and Etiology Toxoplasmosis is the most common cause of posterior segment infections. *Toxoplasma gondii* is an obligate, intracellular parasitic protozoon that is an intestinal parasite in cats. Rodents or birds are intermediate hosts. Humans become infected by ingesting undercooked meat that contains tissue cysts. Until recently, ocular toxoplasmosis was thought to be usually congenital, but acquired disease is more common than previously thought. Episodes may take 3 to 4 months to resolve without treatment.

History Most often a young, healthy adult presents with a recent onset of red eye, photophobia, floaters, and decreased vision.

Important Clinical Signs Focal area of chorioretinal inflammation (Figure 5-2A,B).

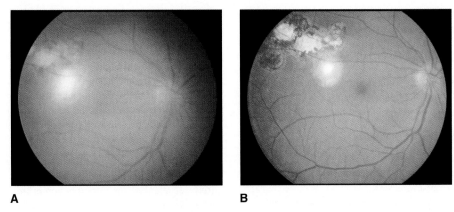

Figure 5-2 Toxoplasmosis chorioretinitis *A. Acute reactivation showing a white, fluffy chorioretinal inflammatory lesion with adjacent pigmentation and overlying vitritis (visual acuity [VA] of 20/300).* **B.** *Same eye after 6 months of treatment with consolidation of the inflammatory focus (VA 20/70).*

Associated Clinical Signs Iritis with large keratic precipitates, intraocular pressure elevation, focal vitreous inflammation directly over the retinal lesion, and vitreous strands coated with inflammatory cells.

Differential Diagnosis

> Other inflammatory chorioretinitis or vitritis (e.g., syphilitic chorioretinitis, sarcoidosis, tuberculosis chorioretinitis)

Diagnostic Evaluation Diagnosis is based on clinical examination and fundus appearance. Serum IgG and IgM antibodies are evaluated for presumed acquired infections. Comparative serology (aqueous versus serum antibodies) is also performed. Polymerase chain reaction (PCR) of the aqueous humor may be useful in atypical cases.

Prognosis and Management

TREATMENT The treatment plan is based on lesion location and severity. Small non–sight-threatening infections can be observed or treated with trimethoprim-sulfamethoxazole or a second-generation tetracycline. Sight-threatening infections such as those near the macula or optic nerve are treated with pyrimethamine, sulfadiazine, and folinic acid. Azithromycin or clindamycin can be used for patients who are allergic to sulfa drugs. The total course of treatment is 5 to 6 weeks. Oral prednisone in low to moderate doses may be used to reduce macular or optic nerve inflammation but should only be given with concurrent antibiotic coverage. Topical steroids and cycloplegic agents are used for anterior segment inflammation.

IMMUNOCOMPROMISED PATIENTS Delays in initiating antibiotic treatment can result in a fulminant course of infection. Ocular toxoplasmosis may present as a multifocal and progressive chorioretinitis simulating cytomegalovirus retinitis and require long-term antibiotics. Neuroimaging to evaluate cerebral toxoplasmosis is suggested.

Ocular Toxocariasis

Definition This entity describes an ocular infection with the nematode *Toxocara canis.*

Epidemiology and Etiology *Toxocara canis* is the intestinal roundworm, found in soil. Systemic signs are not usually seen in children presenting with ocular toxocariasis, but may include visceral larva migrans with eosinophilia, fever, and malaise.

History Children present with unilateral iritis and vitritis accompanied by decreased vision.

Important Clinical Signs Ocular toxocariasis may present as posterior granuloma, peripheral granuloma, or endophthalmitis, with fibrocellular stalks extending to the disc.

Associated Clinical Signs Patients may present with leukokoria. Death of the nematode causes severe inflammation.

Differential Diagnosis

Retinoblastoma
Retinopathy of prematurity
Coats' disease
Persistent hyperplastic primary vitreous
Pars planitis

Diagnostic Evaluation Clinical examination may require examination under anesthesia. Ultrasonography may be needed if intense vitritis is present. *Toxocara* serology may be helpful.

Prognosis and Management Anti-helminthic medications are not required. Intense scar formation may lead to cyclitic membranes and tractional retinal detachment. Vitrectomy surgery and systemic as well as local steroids may be considered.

Cytomegalovirus Retinitis

Definition Cytomegalovirus (CMV) retinitis is a slow-growing herpesvirus infection of the retina and retinal pigment epithelium that occurs in an immunocompromised host.

Epidemiology and Etiology CMV is a double-stranded DNA virus of the herpes family. It is the most commonly seen opportunistic infection in patients with acquired immunodeficiency syndrome (AIDS) and is associated with CD4 (T-helper cell) counts below 50 cells/mm^3. Prior to highly active antiretroviral therapy (HAART), CMV retinitis was a major cause of systemic and ophthalmic morbidity in patients with AIDS. For patients infected with human immunodeficiency virus (HIV) who have CD4 lymphocyte counts below 100, ophthalmic screening every 3 to 6 months is recommended.

History Decreased vision or new onset of floaters is noted in a severely immunocompromised host.

Important Clinical Signs Slowly expanding, full-thickness retinal lesion with a granular, often hemorrhagic border and a central, atrophic portion that develops as the lesion enlarges. Patients usually present with posterior pole disease, although any portion of the retina can be infected (Figure 5-3A–C).

Associated Clinical Signs Mild or absent vitritis, especially in immunocompromised patients. Rhegmatogenous retinal detachment due to retinal holes in atrophic retina may occur at presentation, during reactivation, or in remission. The risk of detachment increases as the area of involvement increases.

Differential Diagnosis

Acute retinal necrosis
Other opportunistic infections (*Pneumocystis carinii*)

Diagnostic Evaluation Based on characteristic clinical examination. Polymerase chain reaction (PCR) on filtered vitreous aspirate and retinal biopsy may be considered for atypical cases of infectious retinitis.

Prognosis and Management (Tables 5-2 and 5-3)

TREATMENT OF INITIAL INFECTIONS Several different treatment regimens are used, as follows: intravenous ganciclovir; intravenous ganciclovir followed by oral ganciclovir; intravenous foscarnet, intravenous cidofovir; intravitreal ganciclovir injections with systemic ganciclovir; or intravitreal ganciclovir implant (Figure 5-3D).

MAINTENANCE THERAPY Consists of oral ganciclovir during remission. With HAART and rising CD4 cell counts, chronic maintenance therapy may not be required, but patients must be cautiously followed.

TREATMENT OF RECURRENT INFECTION Usually requires combination therapy such as intravenous foscarnet and intravenous ganciclovir; cidofovir and intravitreal ganciclovir implant or

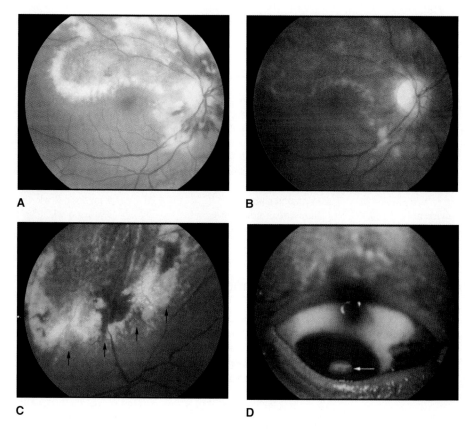

Figure 5-3 Cytomegalovirus (CMV) retinitis *A. Acute CMV retinitis in a patient with acquired immunodeficiency syndrome (AIDS). Hemorrhagic retinal whitening has a predilection for the optic disc and retinal vessels. **B.** Same eye 4 weeks after initiating treatment showing CMV retinitis in remission. **C.** CMV retinitis with active border signified by retinitis and hemorrhage adjacent to atrophic retina (arrows). **D.** Ganciclovir implant (arrow) is noted in the inferior vitreous cavity in an HIV-infected patient with CMV retinitis. Kaposi's sarcoma is noted on the upper eyelid and nasal conjunctiva.*

TABLE 5-2   CYTOMEGALOVIRUS REGIMENS TREATMENT

Drug	Route	Dosage
Ganciclovir	IV induction	5 mg/kg bid × 2 wk
	IV maintenance	5 mg/kg qd
	Oral maintenance	Variable
	Intravitreal injection	2000 μg q wk
	Intravitreal implant	Effective 4–8 mo
Foscarnet	IV induction	60 mg/kg tid × 2–3 wk
	IV maintenance	90–120 mg/kg qd
	Intravitreal injection	1.2 mg in 0.05 mL
Cidofovir	IV induction	5 mg/kg q wk × 2 wk
	IV maintenance	5 mg/kg q 2 wk
Fomivirsen	Intravitreal induction	330 μg q wk × 3 wk
	Intravitreal maintenance	330 μg q 2 wk

IV = intravenous, wk = week.

TABLE 5-3   CYTOMEGALOVIRUS MEDICATION SIDE EFFECTS

Drug	Side Effects
Ganciclovir	Myelosuppression, thrombocytopenia
Foscarnet	Nephrotoxic
Cidofovir	Nephrotoxic, hypotony, uveitis
Fomivirsen	Anterior uveitis, vitritis, increased IOP, cataract

IOP = intraocular pressure.

intravitreal foscarnet; or multiple intravitreal injections. Intravitreal fomivirsen is an antisense compound, consisting of 21 nucleotides, that inhibits virus replication.

RESPONSE TO TREATMENT   Evaluate the size of the lesion using photographs. Determine the degree of activity (retinal whitening, hemorrhage); see Figure 5-3B.

RETINAL DETACHMENT   Managed by pars plana vitrectomy with silicone oil tamponade. Treatment alternatives such as laser demarcation for smaller peripheral detachments can be considered.

Acute Retinal Necrosis

Definition   Acute retinal necrosis (ARN) is a necrotizing herpetic retinitis. Although originally described as a bilateral, confluent, rapidly progressive necrotizing retinitis, initially noted in the periphery and spreading centrally, it may also present unilaterally.

Epidemiology and Etiology   Usually occurs in young, healthy adults. Less common subset populations are elderly patients and immunocompromised patients of any age. Disease is caused by infection of the retina with varicella zoster virus or herpes simplex viruses 1 and 2.

History   A young, healthy adult presents with iritis or episcleritis, and a rapid decline in vision with intense vitritis.

Important Clinical Signs   Vitritis with peripheral retinal whitening (Figure 5-4) that progressively coalesces.

Associated Clinical Signs   Iridocyclitis, intense vitritis, photophobia, optic neuritis, and retinal arteriolitis can be present in the later stages.

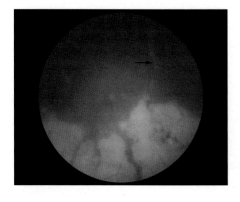

Figure 5-4   Acute retinal necrosis (ARN)
Confluent peripheral retinal whitening and vasculitis (arrow) *with some retinal hemorrhage.*

Differential Diagnosis

CMV retinitis
Pars planitis
Inflammatory chorioretinitis (e.g., Behçet's disease)

Diagnostic Evaluation   Diagnosis is based on clinical examination. Polymerase chain reaction or retinal biopsy may be considered for atypical cases.

Prognosis and Management

LATERALITY   Bilateral involvement on presentation is seen in 20% of patients. The fellow eye may become involved later, usually within 3 months.

SYSTEMIC ANTIVIRAL TREATMENT   This treatment approach is used to reduce the area of retinal damage and perhaps also reduce the rate of involvement of the fellow eye. Antiviral treatment is as follows: at presentation, intravenous acyclovir, 10 mg/kg three times daily for 7 to 10 days, followed by a 3-month course of oral acyclovir (800 mg five times a day) for prophylaxis of the fellow eye.

RETINAL DETACHMENT   Prognosis is dependent on the complication of retinal detachment. The highest risk is 8 to 12 weeks after onset of infection. Demarcation of the lesion borders with laser photocoagulation may decrease the rate of retinal detachment. Surgical repair of retinal detachment by pars plana vitrectomy with silicone oil tamponade may be complicated by hypotony, membrane formation, and postoperative inflammation.

Progressive Outer Retinal Necrosis

Definition   Progressive outer retinal necrosis (PORN) is a devastating, necrotizing herpetic retinitis that affects immunocompromised patients, usually those with AIDS.

Epidemiology and Etiology   Most common in immunocompromised patients. There is a high incidence of bilateral presentation. Caused by herpetic infection of the retina and retinal pigment epithelium (e.g., varicella zoster virus, herpes simplex viruses 1 and 2).

History   Patients commonly have a history of prior herpes zoster dermatitis, such as ipsilateral herpes zoster ophthalmicus, and rapid progression of decreased vision.

Important Clinical Signs   Peripheral or posterior pole outer retinal whitening with rapid circumferential progression (Figure 5-5A–C). There is a characteristic perivascular sparing or "halo" of unaffected retina.

Associated Clinical Signs   Vitritis may be mild or absent.

Differential Diagnosis

CMV retinitis
Inflammatory chorioretinitis
Outer retinal toxoplasmosis

Diagnostic Evaluation   Diagnosis is based on clinical examination. Comparative serology of aqueous humor and serum for varicella IgG antibody and herpes simplex virus IgG

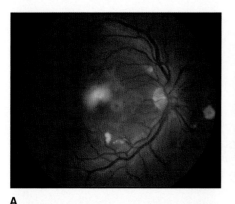

A

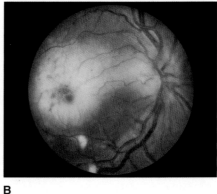

B

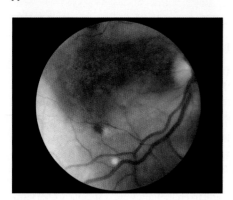

C

Figure 5-5 Progressive outer retinal necrosis (PORN) in a patient with AIDS
*A. Confluent outer retinal whitening in the posterior pole. **B**. Rapidly progressive outer retinal infarction with optic disc involvement over the course of 2 weeks. **C**. Macular necrosis and expanding progressive outer retinal necrosis at 1 to 2 months.*

antibody may be useful. Polymerase chain reaction or retinal biopsy may be considered for atypical cases.

Prognosis and Management Progression to retinal detachment and bilateral blindness is rapid (see Figure 5-5B). Intravenous acyclovir may not be sufficient; therefore, systemic therapy such as ganciclovir or combined therapy of ganciclovir and foscarnet may be used. Intravitreal injections of antiviral agents have also been used to help control the retinitis; however, systemic treatment is still necessary given the known involvement of the central nervous system. Once remission is achieved, intravenous or oral ganciclovir may be sufficient. Visual prognosis is invariably grim.

Syphilitic Chorioretinitis

Definition Infection with *Treponema pallidum* may lead to latent ocular infection manifesting in secondary and tertiary (late) stages of syphilis, as follows:

> *Secondary stage*—6 weeks to 6 months after primary infection, skin rash involving palms, soles, fever, arthralgias
> *Late stage*—disease greater than 1 year after primary infection

Epidemiology and Etiology Sexually transmitted or blood-borne bacterial infection with *Treponema pallidum. Treponema pallidum* is a highly coiled, helical bacteria, referred to as the

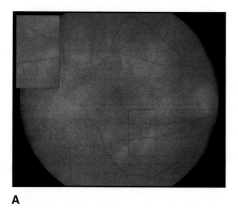
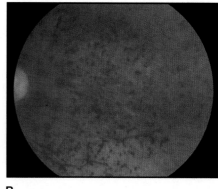

A **B**

Figure 5-6A,B Syphilis *A. Patchy, yellow acute chorioretinitis* (inset) *throughout the macula in a patient with tertiary syphilis.* *B. Syphilitic chorioretinitis with "salt and pepper" pigmentary clumping.*

"great masquerader." Ophthalmic manifestations usually occur in the secondary stage of syphilis.

History Pain, redness, iritis, floaters, and blurred vision are noted in a sexually active patient. Posterior chorioretinitis may be present with a quiet anterior segment.

Important Clinical Signs Active chorioretinitis with yellow, deep infiltrates in the temporal macula (Figure 5-6A) and vitritis. May manifest as a yellow, submacular pseudohypopyon.

Associated Clinical Signs Gummas in the eyelid, orbit, or optic nerve head; stromal keratitis, episcleritis, scleritis, and iridocylitis; retinal vasculitis, optic neuritis, or neuroretinitis. Late sequelae include chorioretinal atrophy and pigmentation, "salt and pepper" fundus with or without vascular narrowing, and optic atrophy (Figure 5-6B).

Differential Diagnosis

Other infectious posterior uveitis
Inflammatory posterior uveitis

Diagnostic Evaluation Variability in presentation justifies evaluation with rapid plasma reagin (RPR) or Venereal Disease Research Laboratory (VDRL) testing for all patients with posterior uveitis; a positive RPR or VDRL is confirmed with fluorescent treponema antibody absorption

(FTA-ABS) or microlhem agglulination-*Treponema pallidum* (MHA-TP) testing. HIV-infected patients may not have a positive RPR or VDRL. VDRL and RPR return to normal with effective therapy.

LATE STAGE DISEASE If the patient has ocular inflammation, neuroophthalmologic findings, HIV infection, or treatment failure, then lumbar puncture should be performed to evaluate for neurosyphilis.

Prognosis and Management

OCULAR SYPHILIS Should be treated as neurosyphilis. Options include:

Penicillin G, 2 to 5 million units IV every 4 hours for 10 to 14 days
Penicillin G procaine, 2 to 4 million units IM every day (with 500 mg probenecid every 4 hours) for 10 to 14 days
For patients allergic to penicillin—doxycycline, 200 mg orally bid for 15 days, or erythromycin, 500 mg orally qid for 15 days

Secondary syphilis responds well to treatment. Tertiary or latent ocular syphilis does not respond well. Topical steroids may be used for anterior uveitis when combined with antibiotic treatment; however, oral steroids usually are not necessary.

Candida **Retinitis**

Definition   This disease is an endogenous fungal infection of the choroid and retina caused by *Candida albicans* or other *Candida* species.

Epidemiology and Etiology   Incidence is increasing owing to use of immunosuppressive treatments, intravenous drugs, and hyperalimentation. An endogenous source for infection can usually be identified. Infection spreads via metastasis to the choroid.

History   Recently hospitalized patients or patients with an indwelling catheter develop decreased vision or floaters. Patients may or may not be immunocompromised.

Important Clinical Signs   In the typical growth pattern, choroidal infiltrate consolidates to form a subretinal nodule that leads to preretinal extension and vitreous seeding. There is a "string-of-pearl" appearance or "headlight-in-a-fog" appearance when the vitritis is significant. (Figure 5-7A–C).

Associated Clinical Signs   Mild to moderate vitritis.

Differential Diagnosis

Inflammatory chorioretinitis

Diagnostic Evaluation   The organism is difficult to culture. Pars plana vitrectomy may be necessary to obtain an adequate sample. Filtration of the vitreous material for culture is necessary.

Prognosis and Management   Infection should be suspected in any patient with uveitis and a potential fungal source. Treatment (Table 5-4) is based on location: for choroidal and subretinal lesions, intravenous amphotericin B or oral azole

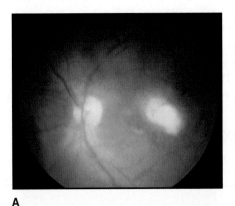

A

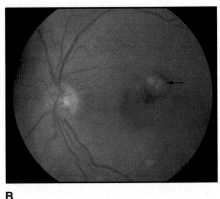

B

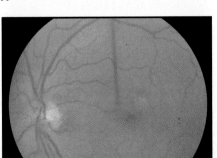

C

Figure 5-7   *Candida* **retinitis**
A. Candida *retinitis: Fluffy, white lesion in the fovea with mild overlying vitritis* (arrow).
B. Candida *chorioretinitis may present with minimal vitreous inflammation and a choroidal granuloma* (arrow). *Note the submacular fluid and intraretinal hemorrhage.*
C. After treatment with systemic antifungal therapy, the granuloma and serous macular detachment has rapidly resolved.

TABLE 5-4　DOSAGE OF MEDICATIONS FOR CANDIDA RETINITIS

Drug	Route	Dosage
Amphotericin B	Intravitreous	5 μg
	Intravenous	25 μg qd; total 1 g
Fluconazole	Intravenous	100–200 mg bid

antifungal drugs are used; for preretinal or vitreous infections, intravitreal amphotericin B. Vitrectomy may be necessary if dense vitritis is present. An infectious disease consultation should be obtained. Use of steroids as a primary agent should be avoided; however, they can be used in combination with effective antifungal therapy.

HIV Retinopathy

Definition　This entity describes retinopathy associated with HIV infection.

Epidemiology and Etiology　HIV retinopathy is the most common ocular finding in patients with AIDS and is present in 50% to 70% of cases. HIV virus has been isolated from the retina, and HIV antigen detected in retinal endothelial cells.

History　The condition affects persons infected with HIV; however, significant presenting symptoms may be absent.

Important Clinical Signs　Retinal hemorrhages, microaneurysms, and cotton-wool spots (Figure 5-8).

Associated Clinical Signs　Anterior uveitis, inflammatory reactions in the vitreous, and chronic multifocal retinal infiltrates.

Differential Diagnosis

　CMV retinitis
　Other opportunistic infections

Diagnostic Evaluation　Diagnosis is based on clinical examination. Photography is helpful to document progression or clearance of lesions.

Prognosis and Management　Findings tend to improve with systemic antiretroviral treatments. No specific ocular treatment is needed.

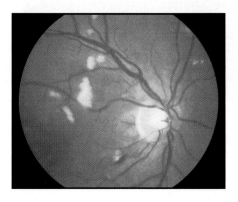

Figure 5-8　HIV retinopathy　*HIV retinopathy in a patient with cotton-wool spots and intraretinal hemorrhages.*

Diffuse Unilateral Subacute Neuroretinitis

Definition Diffuse unilateral subacute neuroretinitis (DUSN) is a unilateral, progressive, widespread, infectious retinitis of parasitic origin.

Epidemiology and Etiology Infection occurs in young patients, probably as a result of fecal-oral contamination. Two sizes of worms produce the same syndrome:

> *Southern United States and Brazil*—small worm of 400 to 1000 μm; possible agents are *Toxocara canis, Ancylostoma caninum* (dog hookworm), *Baylisascaris procyonis* (raccoon)
> *Northern United States*—larger worm of 1500 to 2000 μm; possible agent is *Baylisascaris procyonis*

The likelihood of DUSN is increased in warmer climates due to lack of ground freezing.

History Progressive unilateral loss of vision occurs in a young patient.

Important Clinical Signs Yellow-white focal chorioretinal inflammatory lesions. Successive examinations show migratory pattern of lesions.

Associated Clinical Signs Pigmentary changes, vascular attenuation, optic atrophy, and vitritis (Figure 5-9A,B).

Differential Diagnosis

> Inflammatory retinitis (e.g., syphilitic retinitis, sarcoidosis)

Diagnostic Evaluation Diagnosis is based on clinical examination. Frequent examinations at short-term intervals (with or without fundus photography) may be needed to directly visualize the worm. The electroretinogram is diminished late in the disease.

Prognosis and Management

PROGNOSIS Effective treatment leads to stabilization of active lesions. Vision stabilizes but does not improve.

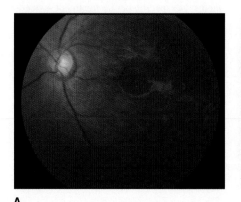

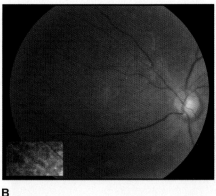

A   B

Figure 5-9 Diffuse unilateral subacute neuroretinitis (DUSN) *A. Posterior pole with mild optic nerve pallor and retinal pigment epithelial alterations. B. Nasal retina with diffuse retinal pigment epithelial changes* (inset).

IDENTIFICATION OF THE NEMATODE Bright lights during examination may cause the nematode to move; once the worm is identified, laser photocoagulation is used to destroy it.

MEDICAL TREATMENT Thiabendazole can be used to kill the worm. A new focal chorioretinal lesion is noted 4 to 7 days after medication. Laser photocoagulation to the new lesion is then used to ensure worm death.

Presumed Ocular Histoplasmosis Syndrome

Definition Presumed ocular histoplasmosis syndrome (POHS) is the term used to describe multifocal, bilateral chorioretinal inflammatory foci caused by the pulmonary pathogen *Histoplasma capsulatum* (soil mold). The classic triad of POHS consists of punched-out chorioretinal scars ("histo spots"), acute or chronic macular exudative changes from choroidal neovascularization, and peripapillary chorioretinal atrophy. The presence of two features in the appropriate clinical setting establishes the diagnosis of POHS.

Epidemiology and Etiology Patients are often between 20 and 50 years of age. Infection is seen most commonly in the Ohio-Mississippi River valley region and southern United States but may be observed in any region. In endemic areas, so-called "histo spots" are noted in approximately 2% to 3% of the population.

History Infection may be asymptomatic or result in decreased vision with or without floaters. The pulmonary infection is typically subclinical.

Important Clinical Signs Multifocal, small yellowish chorioretinal lesions are typically less than 1 mm in size and clustered in the posterior pole, often with pigmentary change (compare with lesions of multifocal choroiditis, which often lack pigment) (Figure 5-10A). Peripapillary pigmentary changes are observed.

There is a lack of vitritis (compare with multifocal choroiditis).

Associated Clinical Signs Macular lesions may be associated with subsequent choroidal neovascularization (Figure 5-10B-D). Chronic, inactive lesions become pigmented and "punched out."

Differential Diagnosis Multifocal choroiditis and other panuveitides such as sarcoidosis, tuberculosis, syphilis, and other "white dot syndromes" should be ruled out. Myopic degeneration may demonstrate peripapillary pigmentary changes.

Diagnostic Evaluation Diagnosis is based on clinical examination. Fluorescein angiography can help differentiate active lesions from choroidal neovascularization.

Prognosis and Management Prognosis depends on the integrity of the macula and whether there are threatening histo spots or choroidal neovascularization. Amsler grid monitoring is used for asymptomatic patients; laser photocoagulation for those with extrafoveal choroidal neovascularization. Photodynamic therapy or submacular surgery is considered for patients with subfoveal choroidal neovascularization.

Multifocal Choroiditis

Definition Multifocal choroiditis describes a condition of idiopathic, multifocal, bilateral chorioretinal inflammatory foci. An infectious etiology has not been confirmed.

Epidemiology and Etiology Disease is more common in women. The etiology is unknown.

History Patients have decreased vision with or without floaters.

Important Clinical Signs Mild vitritis. Multifocal, small yellowish chorioretinal lesions are typically clustered in the posterior pole (Figure 5-10E). Active lesions come and go over time.

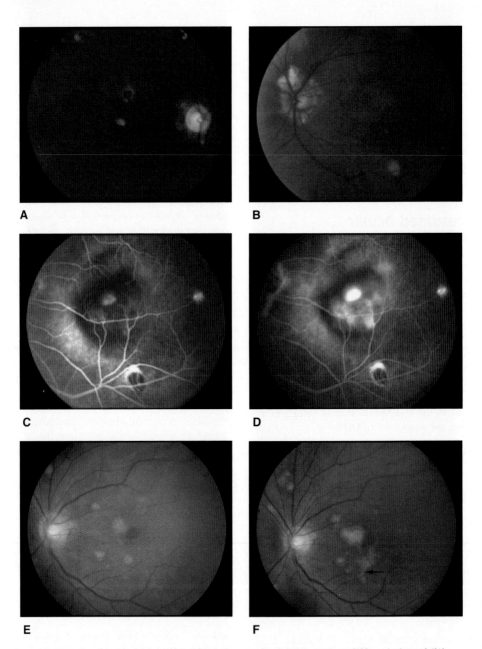

Figure 5-10A–F Presumed ocular histoplasmosis (POHS) and multifocal choroiditis
A. POHS: Peripapillary pigmentary changes and pigmented "histo spots" in the macula.
B. POHS: Patient noted a sudden loss of vision with submacular fluid and pigmented choroidal neovascularization (CNV) near a small histo spot inferior to the fovea. C. POHS: Fluorescein angiogram showing subfoveal CNV and a surrounding area of hypofluorescence. Histo spots show transmission hyperfluorescence. D. POHS: Late-phase fluorescein angiogram showing leakage of dye from CNV. E. Multifocal choroiditis in a 32-year-old healthy woman. Multiple, acute, deep, yellow lesions with active, indistinct borders are seen (VA 20/300). Note the relative lack of pigmentation. F. Multifocal choroiditis: Chronic stage of the same patient as in (E), with inactive lesions and areas of pigmentation (VA 20/70). Note the early bridging subretinal fibrosis (arrow).

Associated Clinical Signs Peripapillary pigmentary changes. Macular lesions may be associated with subsequent choroidal neovascularization. Chronic, inactive lesions become pigmented and "punched out" (Figure 5-10F). A more severe variant of multifocal choroiditis may be associated with subretinal fibrosis and subretinal bridging fibrous bands.

Differential Diagnosis Multifocal choroiditis is a diagnosis of exclusion. Other panuveitides such as sarcoidosis, tuberculosis, syphilis, and other "white dot syndromes" should be ruled out.

Diagnostic Evaluation Diagnosis is based on clinical examination. Fluorescein angiography can help differentiate active lesions from choroidal neovascularization.

Prognosis and Management This is a chronic, recurrent condition. Prognosis depends on macular function (cystoid macular edema, choroidal neovascularization). Oral or sub-Tenon injection of corticosteroids is administered for active macular inflammation. Laser photocoagulation or photodynamic therapy of choroidal neovascularization may be used, depending on location.

NONINFECTIOUS CAUSES

Multiple Evanescent White Dot Syndrome

Definition   Multiple evanescent white dot syndrome (MEWDS) is an idiopathic inflammatory disease of the retina.

Epidemiology and Etiology   Affects myopic individuals, usually between 15 and 47 years of age, as follows: women, 90%; men, 10%.

History   Patients have decreased vision in one eye.

Important Clinical Signs   Unilateral, multiple, small (100 to 200 μm) outer retinal white dots are present in the posterior pole (often subtle) and surrounding the optic disc. "Granular" foveal retinal pigment epithelial alterations are also seen (Figure 5-11A–C).

Associated Clinical Signs   Papillitis with an enlarged blind spot.

Differential Diagnosis

Other "white dot syndromes"

Diagnostic Evaluation   Fluorescein angiography shows characteristic "wreath-like" hyperfluorescent lesions (Figure 5-11B).

Prognosis and Management   Prognosis is good. Lesions usually resolve spontaneously by 6 to 12 weeks. The disease may be recurrent, but it rarely may become sequentially bilateral. No treatment is indicated.

Acute Multifocal Placoid Pigment Epitheliopathy

Definition   Acute multifocal placoid pigment epitheliopathy (AMPPE) is a self-limited, acute, bilateral, multifocal inflammatory condition of the retina and choroid.

Epidemiology and Etiology   Most common in adolescents and young adults. Etiology is unknown.

History   Patients have decreased vision, paracentral scotomas, and a history of prodromal (33%) flu-like illness.

Important Clinical Signs   Multiple, cream-colored, plaque-like lesions are seen deep to the retina. Lesions tend to be large with blurred edges, appear confluent (Figure 5-12A) and are clustered in the posterior pole.

Associated Clinical Signs   Mild anterior chamber and vitreous inflammation; occasionally optic nerve edema. Cerebral vasculitis is a rare, life-threatening complication.

Differential Diagnosis

Other "white dot syndromes"
Serpiginous choroidopathy

Diagnostic Evaluation   Diagnosis is based on clinical examination. Fluorescein angiography shows lesions to have early hypofluorescence and late hyperfluorescence (Figure 5-12B,C).

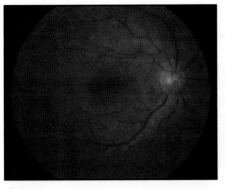

A

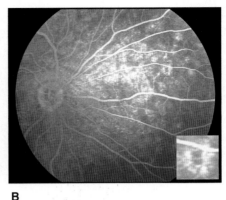

B

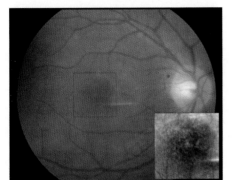

C

Figure 5-11 Multiple evanescent white dot syndrome (MEWDS) *A. Color fundus photo showing multiple, small, uniform, deep yellow lesions, some of which are confluent.* *B. Corresponding fluorescein angiogram showing the spots to have a characteristic "wreath-like" pattern of hyperfluorescence* (inset). *C. Foveal granularity* (inset) *characteristic of MEWDS.*

Prognosis and Management Visual prognosis is usually good, unless the fovea becomes involved. The condition does not usually recur. There is no evidence that steroid treatment is beneficial if the fovea is not affected.

Birdshot Chorioretinitis

Definition Birdshot chorioretinitis describes a bilateral, idiopathic, multifocal chorioretinitis.

Epidemiology and Etiology Most common in patients who are 40 years of age and older.

This idiopathic condition occurs more often in women and is associated with HLA-A29.

History Patients have decreased vision, difficulty with night vision, and impaired color perception.

Important Clinical Signs Multiple, cream-colored, medium-sized lesions at the level of the retinal pigment epithelium. Lesions tend to radiate from the optic nerve like birdshot from a shotgun, hence the name given to the condition (Figure 5-13A,B).

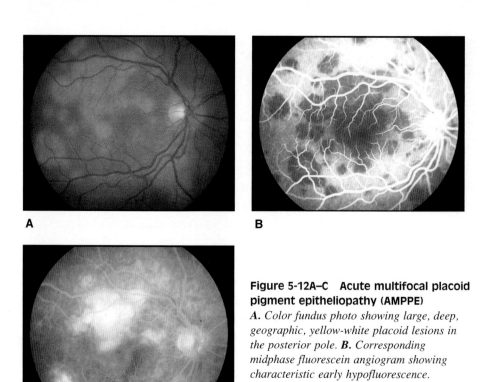

Figure 5-12A–C   Acute multifocal placoid pigment epitheliopathy (AMPPE)
A. Color fundus photo showing large, deep, geographic, yellow-white placoid lesions in the posterior pole. B. Corresponding midphase fluorescein angiogram showing characteristic early hypofluorescence. C. Late-phase fluorescein angiogram demonstrating late hyperfluorescence and submacular fluid.

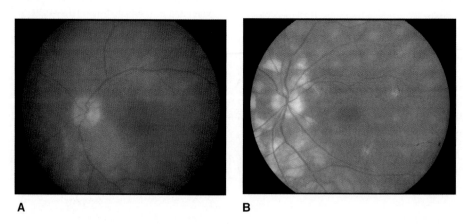

Figure 5-13A,B   Birdshot chorioretinitis   *A. Multiple, subtle, medium-sized, yellow lesions that appear to radiate from the optic nerve. There is mild cystoid macular edema and mild vitritis. This patient is HLA-B27 positive. B. Another patient demonstrating more advanced, atrophic lesions radiating throughout the fundus.*

Associated Clinical Signs Cells in the anterior segment are minimal or absent; mild vitreous cells may be observed; retinal vessels are attenuated and may have sheathing. Disc edema or optic atrophy may be present. Epiretinal membranes and choroidal neovascularization may occur.

Differential Diagnosis

Other "white dot" inflammatory conditions

Diagnostic Evaluation Diagnosis is based on clinical examination. Fluorescein angiography shows perifoveal capillary leakage. Cystoid macular edema is common. The electroretinogram is usually reduced or absent in advanced cases.

Prognosis and Management Oral corticosteroids and immunosuppressive agents have been used with questionable efficacy. Periocular steroids are useful for cystoid macular edema. The condition may respond to cyclosporine. Chronic disease with multiple exacerbations may lead to poor visual prognosis.

Vogt-Koyanagi-Harada Syndrome

Definition Vogt-Koyanagi-Harada (VKH) syndrome describes a bilateral, diffuse, granulomatous uveitis with chorioretinitis that is not associated with previous trauma or surgery.

Epidemiology and Etiology Most common in Asian or American Indians, aged 30 to 50 years. It is associated with HLA-DR4. Etiology is unknown, but may involve an immune reaction to uveal melanin-associated protein.

History Patients have a bilateral decrease in vision, highly variable pain, redness, and photophobia.

Important Clinical Signs Anterior uveitis with keratic precipitates and synechiae. Posterior uveitis with exudative retinal detachment and vitreous cells (Figure 5-14A).

Associated Clinical Signs

OCULAR   Optic neuropathy.

SYSTEMIC   Headache, stiff neck, loss of consciousness, paralysis, seizures, and focal neurologic signs.

SKIN   Alopecia, vitiligo, and poliosis.

Differential Diagnosis

Sympathetic ophthalmia
Posterior scleritis

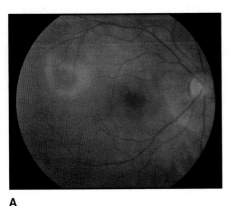
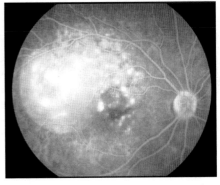

A   **B**

Figure 5-14   Vogt-Koyanagi-Harada (VKH) syndrome *A. Color fundus photo showing exudative serous retinal detachment with deep gray, subretinal lesions. B. Corresponding fluorescein angiogram with multiple pinpoint hyperfluorescent areas, subretinal leakage, and accumulation of dye.*

TABLE 5-5 **DIFFERENTIAL DIAGNOSIS OF FLUORESCEIN ANGIOGRAM DEMONSTRATING MULTIPLE PINPOINT AREAS OF LEAKAGE AT THE LEVEL OF THE RETINAL PIGMENT EPITHELIUM**

Inflammatory	Ischemic	Infiltrative
Vogt-Koyanagi-Harada Syndrome	Malignant hypertension	Leukemia
Posterior scleritis	Toxemia of pregnancy	Lymphoma
Sympathetic ophthalmia		Some choroidal tumors

Diagnostic Evaluation Diagnosis is based on clinical examination. Fluorescein angiography shows multiple, pinpoint, hyperfluorescent dots with leakage of dye (Figure 5-14B, and Table 5-5). Ultrasonography shows diffuse choroidal thickening. Cerebral spinal fluid evaluation shows transient lymphocytosis.

Prognosis and Management

COMPLICATIONS These include secondary glaucoma, choroidal neovascularization, and cataracts.

TREATMENT Systemic, local, or periocular corticosteroids are administered, usually for 3 or more months, and then tapered slowly. Cycloplegic agents are necessary to avoid development of synechiae. Cyclosporine may be considered for patients who are intolerant of or poorly responsive to steroids.

Sympathetic Ophthalmia

Definition Sympathetic ophthalmia is a rare, latent, bilateral nonnecrotizing, granulomatous inflammation that occurs after ocular injury or surgery. "Exciting eye" is used to refer to the traumatized or operated eye; "sympathizing eye" is the fellow eye with latent inflammation (uninjured).

Epidemiology and Etiology

INCIDENCE Significantly decreased due to improved wound closure and early enucleation of severely injured eyes.

ETIOLOGY Unknown; possibly hypersensitivity to pigment or retinal S antigen.

Pathology Diffuse granulomatous uveal involvement, no reaction in the choriocapillaris, epithelioid cells with uveal pigment, and Dalen-Fuchs nodules.

History Patients have had previous ocular trauma or surgery with variable conjunctival injection, photophobia, and decreased vision in the fellow eye.

Important Clinical Signs

INJURED EYE Severe panuveitis.

SYMPATHIZING EYE Large, mutton-fat keratic precipitates; peripheral anterior synechiae; multiple, yellow subretinal lesions (Dalen-Fuchs nodules) (Figure 5-15A); and vitritis.

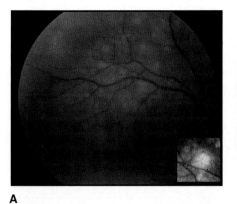

A

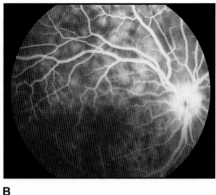

B

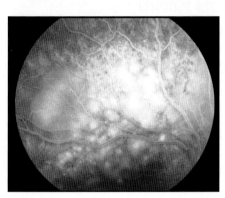

C

Figure 5-15   Sympathetic ophthalmia
A. Color fundus photo showing multiple, deep, yellow subretinal lesions (inset).
B. Midphase fluorescein angiogram with multiple plaque-like areas of hyperfluorescence and optic disc hyperfluorescence.
C. Late-phase fluorescein angiogram with subretinal dye leakage and pooling.

Associated Clinical Signs   An early clinical symptom may be reduced accommodation in the sympathizing eye.

SYMPATHIZING   Papillitis and exudative retinal detachment are also common.

Differential Diagnosis

Other exudative inflammatory diseases such as posterior scleritis or VKH syndrome

Diagnostic Evaluation   Diagnosis is based on clinical history and examination. Fluorescein angiography shows multiple, pinpoint, hyperfluorescent dots with subretinal leakage of dye (Figure 5-15B,C).

Prognosis and Management   Most patients experience a chronic clinical course with frequent flare-ups. An improved prognosis is associated with rapid diagnosis and effective treatment. Local, periocular, or systemic corticosteroids are administered. Antimetabolites, such as cyclosporine, are sometimes needed.

Ocular Sarcoidosis

Definition This term describes ocular manifestations in a patient with sarcoidosis.

Epidemiology and Etiology

EPIDEMIOLOGY More common in African Americans but is observed in all races. Patients are usually between 20 and 50 years old.

SYSTEMIC DISEASE This is a multisystem disease that usually affects pulmonary function but can affect liver, skin, and central nervous system functioning.

Pathology Noncaseating epithelioid cell granuloma, and central areas of fibrinoid degeneration.

History Patients present with blurred vision and aching around the eyes.

Important Clinical Signs Anterior, acute, or chronic, granulomatous iridocyclitis with mutton-fat keratic precipitates; peripheral anterior synechiae; and anterior and posterior vitritis (Figure 5-16A).

Associated Clinical Signs

POSTERIOR INVOLVEMENT Cystoid macular edema; venous sheathing; peripheral chorioretinal white spots; "candle-wax drippings" or irregular nodular granulomas surrounding venules; yellow-grey nodular granulomas of the retina, choroid, and optic nerve; and retinal neovascularization (Figure 5-16B-E).

CUTANEOUS INVOLVEMENT Orbital and eyelid granulomas.

OTHER OCULAR SIGNS Conjunctival granulomas, bulbar and palpebral; iris nodules; cataract; keratitis sicca; and secondary glaucoma.

Differential Diagnosis

Other inflammatory chorioretinal disorders (e.g., syphilis, tuberculosis, toxoplasmosis)

Diagnostic Evaluation Ocular sarcoidosis should be suspected in all patients with uveitis. Evaluation include determination of serum lysozyme and angiotensin-converting enzyme levels; chest X-ray; limited gallium scan of the neck and head; and biopsy of suspicious skin, conjunctival, or lacrimal gland lesions. Fluorescein angiography may show vascular leakage (see Figure 5-16B).

Prognosis and Management Prognosis is variable. Topical, periocular, or systemic steroids and cycloplegia may be used for comfort as well as prevention of synechiae. Systemic antimetabolites such as methotrexate are also sometimes used.

Pars Planitis

Definition Pars planitis is an idiopathic, noninfectious inflammation of the vitreous cavity.

Epidemiology and Etiology Pars planitis is most common in those younger than 40 years, and 80% of cases are bilateral. Etiology is unknown.

History

CHILDREN Patients present with red eye with photophobia and significant inflammation of the anterior segment.

YOUNG ADULTS Patients present with floaters.

Important Clinical Signs Anterior vitritis or posterior vitritis with "snowballs" (aggregates of vitreous cells). "Snowbanking" refers to the aggregation of dense vitritis along the inferior vitreous base and pars plana region (Figure 5-17).

Associated Clinical Signs Posterior synechiae, posterior subcapsular cataract, cystoid macular edema (major cause of visual loss), epiretinal membrane, dense vitritis, vitreous hemorrhage, peripheral neovascularization, and band keratopathy.

Differential Diagnosis

Other causes of vitritis such as sarcoidosis, multiple sclerosis, Lyme disease, toxocariasis, syphilis, and tuberculosis

Diagnostic Evaluation Diagnosis is based on clinical examination. Fluorescein angiography may show retinal venular leakage or cystoid macular edema.

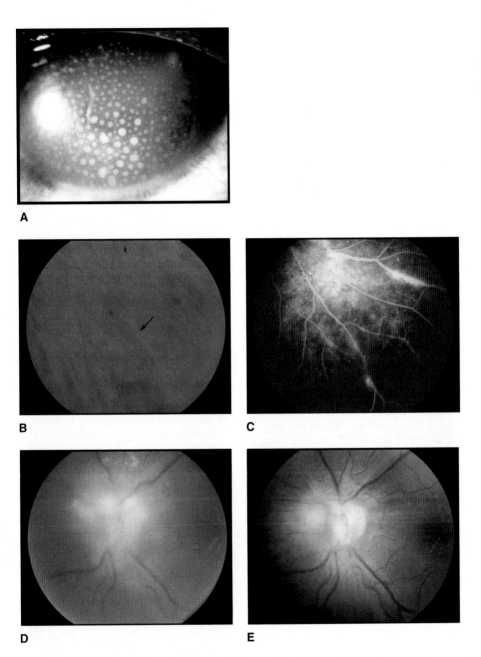

Figure 5-16 Ocular sarcoidosis *A. Mutton-fat keratic precipitates of ocular sarcoidosis.*
B. Color fundus photo of the peripheral retina showing retinal venous sheathing (arrow).
C. Corresponding fluorescein angiogram showing vascular fluorescein staining and mild
leakage. *D. Optic disc granuloma due to sarcoidosis. There is overlying vitritis and macular star*
formation. *E. Partial resolution of the optic disc granuloma is observed 3 months after treatment*
with systemic steroids.

NONINFECTIOUS CAUSES

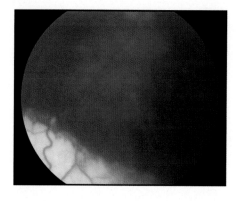

Figure 5-17 Pars planitis *Peripheral retinal and subretinal inflammation extending from inferior "snowbank."*

Prognosis and Management

MEDICAL TREATMENT The therapy varies with the severity of disease and its effect on vision. Patients with normal vision generally do not require treatment. Corticosteroids (administered topically, sub-Tenon, or orally) are used in patients whose vision is decreased. Oral methotrexate, cyclosporine, or cyclophosphamide also may be used.

SURGICAL TREATMENT Patients may require cryoablation of the snowbank. Vitrectomy may be performed for dense vitritis or vitreous hemorrhage or refractory cystoid macular edema.

Behçet's Disease

Definition This entity is an idiopathic, systemic vasculitic condition that involves a classic triad of iritis with hypopyon, stomatitis (aphthous mouth ulcers), and genital ulcers.

Epidemiology and Etiology The disease affects young adults and is more common in the region from the Eastern Mediterranean to Japan. It is often bilateral and is associated with HLA-B5.

History Patients present with the characteristic triad of ocular, oral, and genital symptoms.

Important Ocular Clinical Signs Acute anterior and posterior uveitis with or without hypopyon.

Associated Clinical Signs

POSTERIOR INVOLVEMENT May include retinal vasculitis, hemorrhages, macular edema, focal retinal necrosis, and ischemic optic neuropathy (Figure 5-18).

CONNECTIVE TISSUE FINDINGS Erythema nodosum, recurrent arthralgias, and arthritis.

OTHER FINDINGS Oral and genital ulcers, ulcerative hemorrhages in the gastrointestinal tract, and central nervous system involvement such as stroke and cranial nerve palsies.

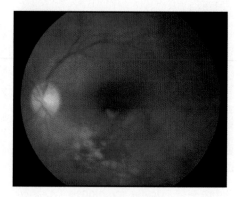

Figure 5-18 Behçet's disease *Localized retinitis with retinal hemorrhages and vascular sheathing. (Reprinted with permission from Regillo CD, Brown GC, Flynn Jr HW. Vitreoretinal Disease: The Essentials 1999, Thieme, New York.)*

Differential Diagnosis

Other inflammatory conditions (e.g., sarcoidosis, syphilis, tuberculosis)

Diagnostic Evaluation Ophthalmic examination and rheumatology consultation are recommended to help establish the diagnosis.

Prognosis and Management This is a chronic, recurring condition that tends to recur typically over a 2- to 4-year period. There is a variable ocular prognosis. Oral corticosteroids are administered, sometimes along with immunosuppressants or other agents such as cyclosporine, chlorambucil, azathioprine, and colchicines.

Serpiginous Chorioretinitis

Definition This entity is a chronic, recurrent inflammation of the choroid, retinal pigment epithelium, and choriocapillaris, which affects the posterior pole in a peripapillary or macular location.

Epidemiology and Etiology The condition is most common in those 40 to 60 years of age, with an equal predilection for sex. Etiology is unknown.

History Patients have blurred vision with a relapsing course.

Important Clinical Signs Map-like pattern of scars in the posterior pole with active edges (yellow-gray and edematous); snake-like pattern of contiguous chorioretinitis in different stages of activity; usually in a peripapillary location (Figure 5-19A,B).

Associated Clinical Signs Mild vitritis, vascular sheathing, and choroidal neovascularization. Optic nerve neovascularization is rare.

Differential Diagnosis

Other inflammatory "white dot syndromes"

Diagnostic Evaluation Diagnosis is based on clinical presentation, ocular examination initially, and indolent course. Fluorescein angiography (Figure 5-19C,D) shows early hypofluorescence and late hyperfluorescence in areas of active chorioretinitis, and "window defect" hyperfluorescence (without staining) in areas of inactive disease.

Prognosis and Management Progressive disease may lead to poor visual prognosis if the fovea is affected; if the fovea is not affected, visual acuity may be good. Corticosteroids or other immunosuppressive agents (cyclosporine) are used.

Posterior Scleritis

Definition This term describes an inflammation of the posterior sclera.

Epidemiology and Etiology Women are affected more often than men. Inflammation is often unilateral and usually is not associated with any underlying systemic immunologic disorder.

History Patients have a gradual onset of eye pain and decreased vision.

Important Clinical Signs Pain, often boring and deep, and decreased vision.

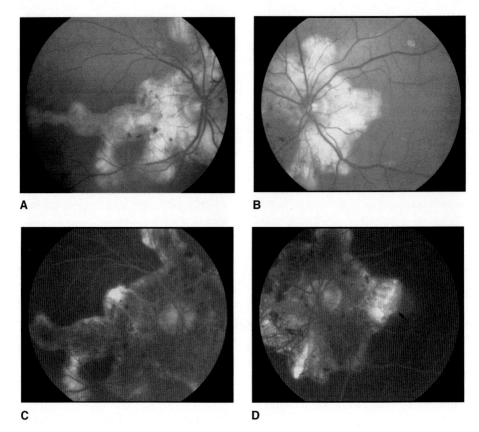

Figure 5-19A-D   Serpiginous choroidopathy in a 46-year-old man with acute visual changes in the right eye   *Color fundus photos of right (A) and left (B) eyes showing peripapillary, snake-like, chorioretinal scarring. Corresponding fluorescein angiogram photographs of right (C) and left (D) eyes revealing diffuse staining of the lesions and an active area with more intense hyperfluorescence at the foveal border in the left eye* (arrow).

Associated Clinical Signs   Choroidal folds, exudative retinal detachment (Figure 5-20A–C), papilledema; angle-closure glaucoma (due to choroidal-scleral thickening), proptosis, and restricted motility are rare.

Differential Diagnosis

Other exudative choroidopathies such as VKH syndrome and sympathetic ophthalmia

Diagnostic Evaluation   Diagnosis is based on clinical examination. Ultrasonography shows thickened posterior sclera, optic nerve "T-sign" (fluid in the posterior sub-Tenon's space) (Figure 5-20D). Fluorescein angiography often shows subretinal leakage of dye.

Prognosis and Management   There is a variable visual prognosis. Treatment consists of oral corticosteroids.

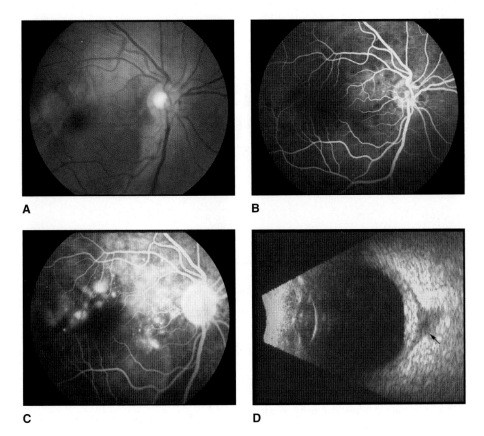

Figure 5-20   Posterior scleritis   *A. Patient presenting with deep, boring eye pain and a serous macular detachment. **B.** Early to midphase fluorescein angiogram showing predominantly patchy hypofluorescence in the posterior pole. **C.** Late-phase fluorescein angiogram demonstrating multiple areas of pinpoint leakage and optic disc hyperfluorescence. **D.** B-scan ultrasound image showing choroidal-scleral thickening with fluid in Tenon's space—the so-called T-sign (arrow).*

Chapter 6

RETINAL DEGENERATIONS AND DYSTROPHIES

Mithlesh Sharma, MD

Allen C. Ho, MD

BEST'S DISEASE

Definition

Best's disease is a macular dystrophy that is clinically characterized by an egg yolk–like lesion at the level of the retinal pigment epithelium (RPE), usually located in the posterior pole. The disease progresses through various stages to culminate in macular atrophy or scarring with loss of central vision.

Synonym—vitelliform macular dystrophy.

Epidemiology and Etiology

Onset Symptoms develop in infancy or early childhood.

Etiology An excessive amount of lipofuscin-like material within the retinal pigment epithelial cells, particularly in the fovea, is observed. There appears be to a secondary loss of the photoreceptor cells.

Genetics It is an autosomal-dominant disease whose gene is mapped to chromosome 11q13.

Clinical Signs

Five stages are delineated:

1. *Previtelliform stage*—patients are asymptomatic with no fundus abnormality, but electrooculography shows a reduced light-peak to dark-trough ratio.
2. *Vitelliform* stage—this stage is characterized by an egg yolk–like lesion in the macular area. It is usually detected during the first or second decade of life. Although usually single and bilaterally symmetric, multiple egg yolk lesions may be observed in the posterior pole. The egg yolk lesions are located at the level of the RPE, are rounded or oval in shape with distinct borders, and range from one-half to two disc diameters in size. Vision may be normal or slightly decreased at this stage (Figure 6-1A,B).
3. *Pseudohypopyon stage*—by the second or third decade of life, lesions break through the RPE, and the yellow material accumulates inferiorly in the macula within the subretinal space to form pseudohypopyon (Figure 6-2A,B).

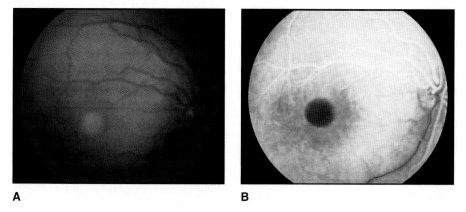

Figure 6-1 Best's disease, vitelliform stage *A. Characteristic egg yolk–like lesion in the fovea.* ***B.*** *Corresponding fluorescein angiogram showing blocked fluorescence due to egg yolk lesion during transit phase. (Courtesy of Retina Slide Collection, Wills Eye Hospital, Philadelphia, Pennsylvania, compiled by Dr. Tamara Vrabec and Dr. Gordon Byrnes.)*

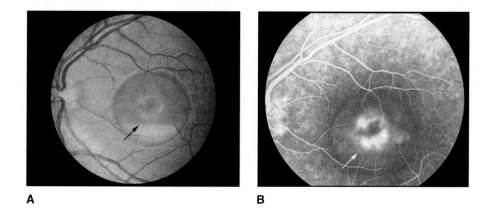

Figure 6-2 Best's disease, pseudohypopyon stage *A. Collection of yellow material within the subretinal space simulating hypopyon* (arrow). ***B.*** *Blocked fluorescence* (arrow) *due to deposition of yellow material inferiorly and perifoveal hyperfluorescence in the center of the lesion is seen in fluorescein angiogram photographs. (Courtesy of Retina Slide Collection, Wills Eye Hospital, Philadelphia, Pennsylvania, compiled by Dr. Tamara Vrabec and Dr. Gordon Byrnes.)*

4. *Vitelliruptive stage*—the egg yolk breaks up to produce a scrambled egg appearance. Patients usually notice some visual impairment at this stage (Figure 6-3A,B).

5. *End stage*—subretinal fibrosis, or a vascularized scar with choroidal neovascularization, contributes to the visual loss at this stage.

The vitelliform degeneration presenting after childhood is called adult Best's disease. In the latter variant, the yellow foveal deposits are symmetric and similar to childhood Best's disease except that the lesions are smaller and have a central pigmented spot. The most common lesion mistaken for Best's disease is a yellow premacular hemorrhage (Figure 6-4A,B).

Diagnostic Evaluation

Visual Acuity   Vision remains good while the egg yolk lesions are intact. Disruption or scarring of the lesions may reduce visual acuity to the level of 20/200.

Visual Fields   Central visual fields are normal initially, but a relative scotoma may develop with time.

Color Vision   Mild dyschromatopsia may be noticed.

Dark Adaptometry   Normal.

Electroretinography   Normal.

Electrooculography   Best's disease is one of the few conditions that result in an abnormal electrooculogram (EOG) in the setting of a normal electroretinogram (ERG). During an EOG, the light-peak:dark-trough ratio (Arden ratio) is typically below 1.5.

Fluorescein Angiography   In the vitelliform stage, complete blockage of background choroidal fluorescence by the lesion is observed. Areas of hyperfluorescence due to atrophic RPE are noticed as the egg yolk lesions show disruption.

Prognosis and Management

In general, the overall prognosis is good as most patients retain reading level of vision in at least one eye throughout life. When severe vision loss does take place in an eye, it occurs slowly and usually begins after the age of 40 years. No treatment is available for Best's disease.

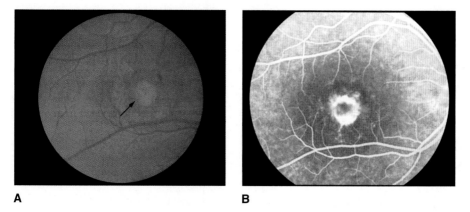

A   **B**

Figure 6-3   Best's disease, vitelliruptive stage   *A. Irregular areas of retinal pigment epithelial loss secondary to breakup of the egg yolk lesion (arrow). **B.** Intense perifoveal hyperfluorescence surrounded by multiple areas of hyperfluorescence is shown in the corresponding fluorescein angiogram. (Courtesy of Retina Slide Collection, Wills Eye Hospital, Philadelphia, Pennsylvania, compiled by Dr. Tamara Vrabec and Dr. Gordon Byrnes.)*

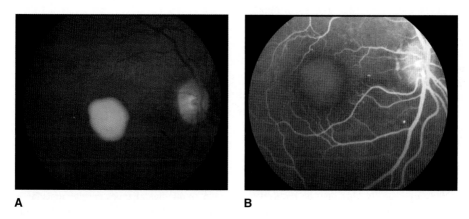

A   **B**

Figure 6-4   Pseudo–Best's disease   *A. Old premacular hemorrhage simulating the egg yolk lesion of Best's disease. Note that the retinal vessels are obscured by the preretinal lesion (arrow). Slightly irregular borders of the lesion and presence of neighboring retinal hemorrhages are clues to the yellow lesion being an old hemorrhage. **B.** Fluorescein angiogram demonstrating microaneurysms and retinal telangiectasia temporal to the lesion, consistent with diabetic retinopathy and a premacular hemorrhage.*

CONE DYSTROPHY

Definition

Cone dystrophy is an inherited defect that primarily affects the cone photoreceptor system.

Epidemiology and Etiology

Onset Symptoms begin in early childhood to middle adulthood.

Genetics Cone dystrophy is primarily autosomal dominant, although autosomal-recessive and X-linked forms have also been reported.

History

The rate of progression and the severity of signs and symptoms are variable. The symptoms consist of progressive visual loss, hemeralopia (decreased vision in brightly illuminated environment), color vision difficulties, and central visual field defects. Macular changes typically follow the visual disturbances; therefore, early in the disease process the fundus may appear entirely normal.

Clinical Signs

Visual Acuity There is gradual, typically symmetric loss of visual acuity to the level of 20/200. Occasionally, this may be reduced to the level of counting fingers to hand motion acuity.

Fundus Changes Variable (Figure 6-5A–D). Early in the disease process, pigmentary stippling with diffuse pigment granularity in the posterior pole is the most common abnormality observed. The classic "bull's-eye" pattern of retinal pigment epithelial atrophy is a late finding. In advanced cases, a round, discrete area of central atrophy is seen. Temporal pallor of the optic disc may be observed.

Differential Diagnosis

Reduced vision with normal fundus in children—in this category, cone dystrophy should be differentiated from Stargardt's disease.

"Bull's-eye" maculopathy—the following causes of "bull's-eye" maculopathy need to be considered in the differential diagnosis:

Stargardt's disease
Chloroquine toxicity
Batten's disease
Benign concentric annular macular dystrophy
Leber's congenital amaurosis

Diagnostic Evaluation

Visual Fields Central scotoma is usually seen.

Color Vision Reduced.

Dark Adaptometry The cone component of the dark adaptation curve is abnormal.

Electroretinography The single-flash photopic ERG and the photopic flicker ERG are low or unrecordable. The scotopic ERG is usually normal.

Fluorescein Angiography The retinal pigment epithelial changes in the macular area may be visible by fluorescein angiography before they can be visualized clinically. Early in the disease process, a mottled hyperfluorescence is seen. As the "bull's-eye" pattern of retinal pigment epithelial loss develops, hyperfluorescence surrounding a central area of hypofluorescence is observed.

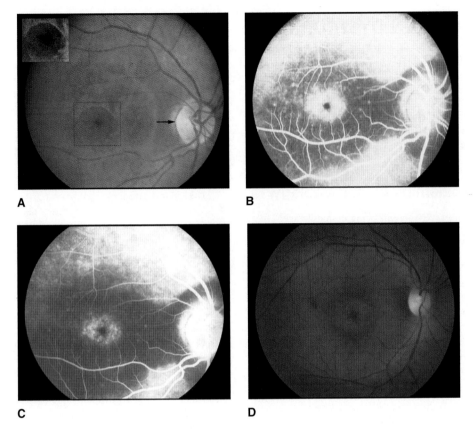

A

B

C

D

Figure 6-5   Cone dystrophy   *A. Early "bull's-eye" maculopathy in a patient with cone dystrophy (inset). Note the temporal optic disc atrophy (arrow). **B.** Corresponding fluorescein angiogram showing central hypofluorescence surrounded by a ring of hyperfluorescence seen during the transit phase (box). **C.** The hyperfluorescence fades away in the later frame indicating the presence of window defects due to retinal pigment epithelial atrophy. **D.** Advanced cone dystrophy with a classic "bull's-eye" maculopathy. Note the temporal optic disc pallor. (Courtesy of Dr. Joseph Maguire and the Retina Slide Collection, Wills Eye Hospital, Philadelphia, Pennsylvania, compiled by Dr. Tamara Vrabec and Dr. Gordon Byrnes.)*

Prognosis and Management

The visual loss is gradual and symmetric to the level of 20/200. However, it may occasionally be severe enough to cause a visual acuity of counting fingers to hand motion. The visual loss is more severe in early-onset cases. No treatment is available for cone dystrophy.

PATTERN DYSTROPHY

Definition

Pattern dystrophy describes a group of related conditions that are inherited in an autosomal-dominant fashion and are clinically characterized by variably shaped yellow or grey deposits in the macula.

Epidemiology and Etiology

Onset Symptoms being in middle age.

Genetics The disease has an autosomal-dominant pattern. Genetic analysis of patients with butterfly dystrophy has shown mutation in the peripherin/RDS gene, located on the short arm of chromosome 6. The peripherin gene product plays an important role in the structural integrity of photoreceptor outer segment discs. However, this mutation does not correspond to a particular phenotype. That is, other forms of retinal degeneration have been linked to peripherin/RDS gene mutations.

History

The majority of patients are either asymptomatic or have minimal visual disturbances. Typically, the diagnosis is made on routine fundus examination of a middle-aged adult.

Clinical Signs

Visual Acuity Patients may have normal visual acuity up to the fifth or sixth decade of life. Reduced vision and metamorphopsia may be the presenting symptoms.

Ophthalmoscopically The following patterns of pigment deposits in the macular area may be observed:

1. Most commonly, a bilateral, triradiate ("butterfly") pattern of yellow or grey pigment at the level of the RPE in the central macular region. A rim of retinal pigment epithelial atrophy around the pigment figure, which is more apparent on fluorescein angiography, may also be seen (Figures 6-6A–C and 6-7A,B).
2. A single, round, vitelliform lesion in the fovea (adult-onset foveomacular vitelliform dystrophy).
3. Extensive macular fishnet arrangement (reticular dystrophy).
4. Coarse pigment mottling of the macula (fundus pulverulentus) (Figure 6-8A,B).

The affected members of a given pedigree may have different patterns, and the patterns may differ in the two eyes of an affected individual. Even a change from one to another pattern over time may be observed.

Differential Diagnosis

Large drusen—ophthalmoscopically, the yellow pigment figures of pattern dystrophy may be confused with the large drusen of age-related macular degeneration.

Diagnostic Evaluation

Visual Fields Normal, except for minimally reduced sensitivity in the macular area.

Color Vision, Dark Adaptometry, Electroretinography Normal.

Electrooculography Mildly abnormal, which is consistent with the disturbed retinal pigment epithelial function.

Fluorescein Angiography Pigment figures are hypofluorescent throughout the study. The retinal pigment epithelial atrophy around the lesions produces hyperfluorescence.

Prognosis

The prognosis for retention of good central vision in at least one eye throughout life is excellent.

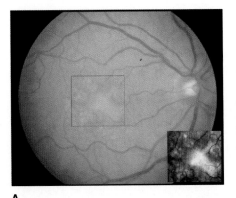

A

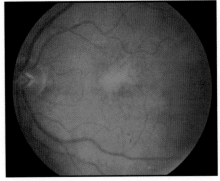

B

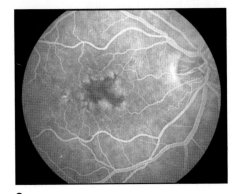

C

Figure 6-6   Pattern dystrophy

A,B. Bilateral, multiple, discrete, yellow areas at the level of the retinal pigment epithelium (RPE) in the central macular region (inset). C. The lesions are more pronounced in the corresponding fluorescein angiogram image of the right eye, where there is patchy hyperfluorescence.

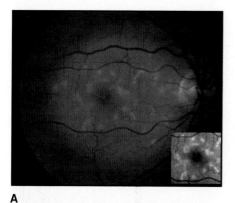

A

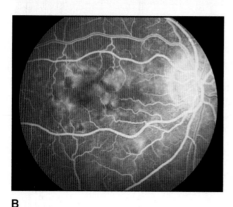

B

Figure 6-7 Pattern dystrophy

A. Classic triradiate ("butterfly") pattern of pigment deposits at the fovea (inset) *surrounded by multiple areas of retinal pigment epithelial atrophy. **B.** Fluorescein angiogram showing patchy hyperfluorescence in the arteriovenous phase. The hyperfluorescent areas correspond to retinal pigment epithelial atrophy in the macular region. (Courtesy of Dr. Eric Shakin and the Retina Slide Collection, Wills Eye Hospital, Philadelphia, Pennsylvania, compiled by Dr. Tamara Vrabec and Dr. Gordon Byrnes.)*

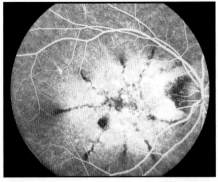

A

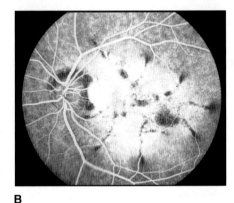

B

Figure 6-8 Pattern dystrophy, fundus pulverulentus *A,B. Fluorescein angiogram photographs of both eyes showing radiating pattern of hypofluorescence due to coarse pigment deposits at the level of RPE— reticular dystrophy. (Courtesy of Dr. William Annesley, and the Retina Slide Collection, Wills Eye Hospital, Philadelphia, Pennsylvania, compiled by Dr. Tamara Vrabec and Dr. Gordon Byrnes.)*

STARGARDT'S DISEASE

Definition

Stargardt's disease is a macular dystrophy that is characterized by the presence of discrete, yellow, pisciform flecks at the level of the RPE. Currently, Stargardt's disease and fundus flavimaculatus are regarded as variants of the same disorder. The term *fundus flavimaculatus* is generally applied when the characteristic flecks are scattered throughout the fundus. When the flecks are confined to the posterior pole and are associated with macular atrophy, the condition is described as Stargardt's disease.

Epidemiology and Etiology

Age The disease usually presents in the first or second decade of life.

Sex Both sexes are affected equally.

Genetics Stargardt's disease is usually autosomal recessive, although dominantly inherited cases have been described. The gene for autosomal-recessive Stargardt's disease is located on chromosome 1. This gene codes for an ATP-binding transport protein (ABCR) that is expressed in the rod inner segments, but not the RPE. A homozygous mutation in the ABCR gene causes fundus flavimaculatus.

History

Children with Stargardt's disease are usually brought to the attention of an ophthalmologist as a result of a gradual impairment of vision noticed by the parents or after failing a school vision screening.

Clinical Signs

Visual acuity is slightly affected in the beginning but may be severely reduced in the later stage of disease. Loss of the foveal reflex may be the only initial clinical finding. Discrete, yellowish, "pisciform" flecks located at the level of the RPE are often noticed at some point in the course of disease. The flecks may or may not involve the macula (Figure 6-9A,B). Perifoveal retinal pigment epithelial mottling may become evident with the progression of disease.

A "bull's-eye" pattern of retinal pigment epithelial loss may become apparent, particularly by fluorescein angiography. The macula classically develops a "beaten bronze" appearance corresponding to atrophy of the central RPE in the advanced stage of disease (Figures 6-10A–C and 6-11A,B). Histopathology shows an accumulation of an abnormal lipofuscin-like material in the RPE (Figure 6-12).

Differential Diagnosis

> *Cone dystrophy*—reduced vision and normal fundus in a child
> *"Bull's-eye" maculopathy*—chloroquine toxicity, Batten's disease, benign concentric annular macular dystrophy

Diagnostic Evaluation

Visual Fields Usually a central scotoma is noted, but a paracentral scotoma, central constriction, and a ring scotoma may also be seen, especially early in the disease.

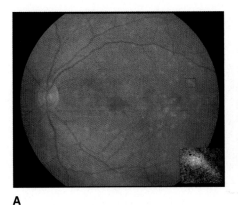
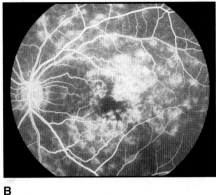

A   **B**

Figure 6-9   Stargardt's disease   *A. Multiple, discrete, yellow, "pisciform" flecks (*inset *shows one fleck) located at the level of the RPE with corresponding hyperfluorescent areas in the fluorescein angiogram photograph are distributed throughout the posterior pole of the left eye. B. The background choroid is dark on the fluorescein angiogram photograph, and there is transmission hyperfluorescence associated with macular flecks and retinal pigment epithelial alterations. (Courtesy of Retina Slide Collection, Wills Eye Hospital, Philadelphia, Pennsylvania, compiled by Dr. Tamara Vrabec and Dr. Gordon Byrnes.)*

Color Vision   Mild dyschromatopsia to red and green may be noted.

Dark Adaptometry   Dark adaptation may be delayed.

Fluorescein Angiography   Features that may help confirm the diagnosis of Stargardt's disease include dark or silent choroid; multiple, irregular hyperfluorescent spots that do not precisely correspond to the flecks; and a "bull's-eye" window-defect pattern of hyperfluorescence in the macula.

Electroretinography   Usually normal but may be reduced with increasing amounts of peripheral flecks and atrophy.

Electrooculography   Usually subnormal.

Prognosis and Management

The majority of patients preserve moderate visual acuity (20/70 to 20/200), at least in one eye. No effective treatment is available for Stargardt's disease.

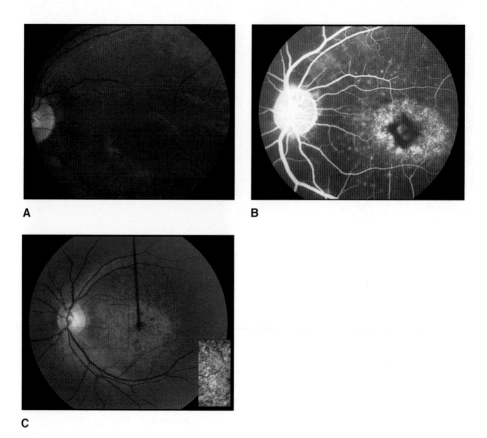

A

B

C

Figure 6-10 Stargardt's disease *A. Advanced Stargardt's disease with "beaten bronze" macula. **B.** Corresponding fluorescein angiogram showing a central area of hypofluorescence (retinal pigment epithelial clumping) surrounded by a ring of hyperfluorescence (retinal pigment epithelial atrophy). Note the dark or silent choroid (blocked fluorescence). **C.** Stargardt's disease with "bull's-eye" macula. Compare with **Figure 6-5D.** Note the "beaten bronze" appearance of the macula (inset). (Courtesy of Dr. Eric Shakin and the Retina Slide Collection, Wills Eye Hospital, Philadelphia, Pennsylvania, compiled by Dr. Tamara Vrabec and Dr. Gordon Byrnes.)*

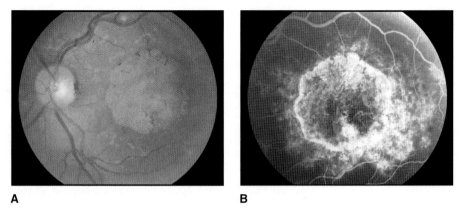

A **B**

Figure 6-11 Stargardt's disease *A. Severe loss of RPE in a geographic fashion in the central macular region in a patient with advanced Stargardt's disease. The visual acuity was reduced to 20/200. **B.** Corresponding fluorescein angiogram showing irregularly distributed areas of hypofluorescence and hyperfluorescence, with a discrete rim of hyperfluorescence within the area of geographic pattern of retinal pigment epithelial loss. Dark choroid is apparent beyond the macula.*

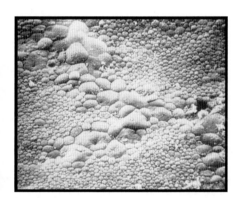

Figure 6-12 Stargardt's disease, electron microphotograph *Electron microphotograph showing enlarged retinal pigment epithelial cells due to intracellular accumulation of lipofuscin-like material. (Courtesy of Dr. Ralph Eagle, Wills Eye Hospital, Philadelphia, Pennsylvania.)*

CHOROIDEREMIA

Definition

Choroideremia is a generalized hereditary retinal degeneration that primarily affects the choriocapillaris and the RPE-photoreceptor complex.

Epidemiology and Etiology

Onset   Symptoms are usually noted in the first or second decade of life.

Sex   Only males are affected, and females are carriers.

Genetics   Choroideremia is an X-linked recessive disorder.

History

Patients usually present in the first or second decade of life with a chief complaint of difficulty with night vision.

Clinical Signs

Early in the disease process, fundus appearance in the affected males is a "salt-and-pepper" retinal pigment epithelial mottling at the equator and the posterior pole. Below the retinal pigment epithelial mottling, the underlying choroid may appear clinically normal, but fluorescein angiography may show a patchy loss of choroidal vasculature.

Later in the disease process, small areas of the RPE drop out in the midperiphery. These areas of drop-out eventually coalesce and progress centrally. The macula is involved last (Figure 6-13A,B). In the final stages, the entire fundus, with an exception of the macula, shows the diffuse yellow-white reflex of the underlying sclera.

Female carriers show unique and pathognomonic fundus features. The generalized retinal pigment epithelial mottling, especially in the midperiphery, resembles the changes seen in males in the early stage of disease. The fundus changes in female carriers remain stationary, and the fluorescein angiography reveals an intact choroidal vasculature.

Differential Diagnosis

Retinitis pigmentosa—unlike retinitis pigmentosa, in choroideremia a "bone-spicule" pattern of pigmentary change is usually not seen, and the retinal blood vessels remain relatively normal.

Gyrate atrophy—in the final stages, fundus appearance in choroideremia may resemble gyrate atrophy, but the different mode of genetic transmission is an important distinguishing feature.

Diagnostic Evaluation

Visual Fields   There is a loss of peripheral visual field.

Electroretinography   This may be normal during the early stage, but by the end of the first decade the scotopic ERG becomes nonrecordable and the photopic ERG is severely reduced.

Fluorescein Angiography   In the early stage, despite the clinically normal appearing choroid, fluorescein angiography may reveal a patchy loss of choriocapillaris. Later in the disease, an extensive loss of choroidal vasculature is observed (Figures 6-14A,B and 6-15A,B).

Prognosis and Management

Relatively good central vision is preserved until late in the disease because the macula is affected late. Although the rate of progression may vary within a pedigree, the majority of patients usually have severely reduced vision by the age of 35 years. Female carriers usually retain normal visual function throughout their life. No treatment is available for choroideremia.

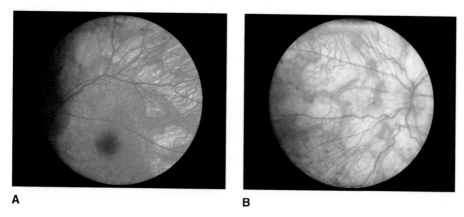

A **B**

Figure 6-13 Choroideremia *A,B. Multiple areas of retinal pigment epithelial loss, some of which have coalesced to form larger patches. Note that the fovea is spared and the patient had 20/40 vision in this eye. (Courtesy of Retina Slide Collection, Wills Eye Hospital, Philadelphia, Pennsylvania, compiled by Dr. Tamara Vrabec and Dr. Gordon Byrnes.)*

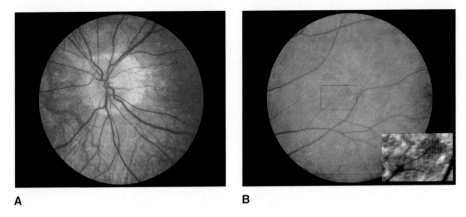

Figure 6-14 Early choroideremia *Peripapillary loss of the RPE (**A**) and subtle pigmentary mottling in the midperipheral fundus (**B**) can be seen* (inset). *Similar fundus findings can be observed in female carriers of choroideremia. (Courtesy of Retina Slide Collection, Wills Eye Hospital, Philadelphia, Pennsylvania, compiled by Dr. Tamara Vrabec and Dr. Gordon Byrnes.)*

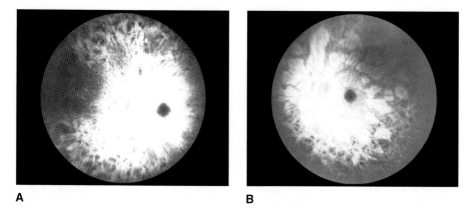

A   **B**

Figure 6-15   **Late choroideremia**   *A. Extensive loss of choriocapillaris is evident in the corresponding late-phase fluorescein angiogram photograph (same patient as **Figure 6-13A**). B. Equator-plus red-free fundus photograph showing multiple patches of the retinal pigment epithelial loss extending from the posterior pole to the midperiphery (same patient as **Figure 6-13B**). (Courtesy of Retina Slide Collection, Wills Eye Hospital, Philadelphia, Pennsylvania, compiled by Dr. Tamara Vrabec and Dr. Gordon Byrnes.)*

GYRATE ATROPHY

Definition

Gyrate atrophy is a rare choroidal disorder, which is usually transmitted in an autosomal-recessive fashion and is caused by an absence or near-absence of the pyridoxine-dependent mitochondrial matrix enzyme ornithine amino-transferase.

Epidemiology and Etiology

Onset Symptoms begin in the first decade of life.

Genetics The disorder is autosomal recessive.

Etiology Elevated levels of ornithine in the plasma and urine in patients with gyrate atrophy are caused by an absence or near-absence of the pyridoxine-dependent mitochondrial matrix enzyme ornithine aminotransferase. The latter is necessary for the breakdown of excess ornithine in humans.

History

The usual presenting symptoms are poor night vision and constricted visual fields.

Clinical Signs

Early in the disease, a thinning and transparency of the RPE, beginning in the midperiphery, is observed. The underlying choroid may appear either normal or sclerotic. The affected areas are separated from the normal-appearing retina by scalloped borders. The involved areas begin as isolated patches but later coalesce (Figure 6-16A–D).

Progression of the disease is accompanied by pigment clumping and choroidal atrophy. Eventually the entire choroidal vasculature disappears, exposing the white sclera. The optic disc and the retinal vessels may be normal early

in the disease, but with time blood vessels show a gradual narrowing.

In the late stages, marked choroidal atrophy from the periphery to the posterior pole is evident. However, the macula is usually spared. Macular involvement may be in the form of macular edema or related to progression of atrophic changes.

Associated Clinical Signs

Ocular

Myopia—almost invariably present
Cataract—seen in a high proportion of patients with gyrate atrophy

Systemic

Characteristically thin, sparse, straight hair
Less consistent findings—abnormal electroencephalogram, muscle weakness, abnormal electrocardiogram, and seizures

Differential Diagnosis

Choroideremia—in late stages, fundus appearance of choroideremia and gyrate atrophy can be remarkably similar. However, different modes of genetic transmission and the distinctive fundus features in the female carriers of choroideremia are important distinguishing features.

Diagnostic Evaluation

Visual Fields Constriction of the peripheral visual fields corresponds to the expansion of the fundus changes.

Fluorescein Angiography A loss of choriocapillaris is demonstrated in the affected areas.

Electroretinography Severely diminished or abolished amplitudes.

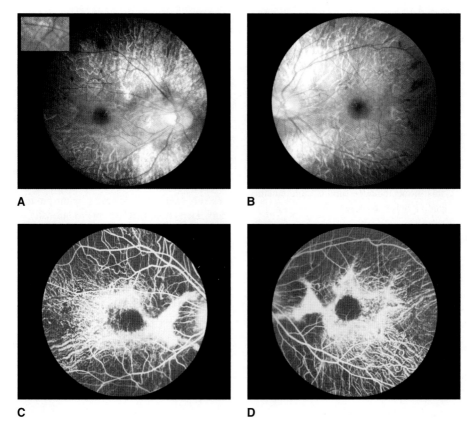

A

B

C

D

Figure 6-16 Gyrate atrophy *A. Bilateral, multiple, geographic patches of retinal pigment epithelial loss with scalloped borders* (inset) *are present in the posterior pole and the peripapillary area.* ***B.*** *Scattered pigmentary clumping is also visible.* ***C,D.*** *Extensive atrophy of the RPE and the choroidal vasculature is evident in the corresponding fluorescein angiogram photographs. The fovea is spared in both eyes, and the patient's visual acuity was 20/40 OD, 20/30 OS. (Courtesy of Retina Slide Collection, Wills Eye Hospital, Philadelphia, Pennsylvania, compiled by Dr. Tamara Vrabec and Dr. Gordon Byrnes.)*

Electrooculography   Abnormal.

Other   Elevated serum ornithine levels and markedly decreased ornithine aminotransferase activity in cultured fibroblasts or leukocytes.

Prognosis and Management

Patients are usually legally blind by the fourth to seventh decade of life. However, earlier visual loss may result from cataract.

Pyridoxine (vitamin B_6) may help normalize the plasma and urinary ornithine levels and preserve visual function. Based on a response to vitamin B_6, gyrate atrophy may have two clinically different subtypes. Patients responsive to vitamin B_6 usually have a less severe and more slowly progressive clinical course than patients who are not responsive. A low-protein diet, particularly a low-arginine diet, may also be of benefit.

CONGENITAL STATIONARY NIGHT BLINDNESS

Congenital stationary night blindness (CSNB) is a group of disorders that is characterized by defective night vision, which remains stable throughout life.

Classification

CSNB with normal fundus appearance.
CSNB with abnormal fundus appearance— this group includes fundus albipunctatus and Oguchi's disease

Fundus Albipunctatus

Definition Fundus albipunctatus (FA) is a disorder of the visual pigment regeneration process that is characterized by an abnormally prolonged recovery of normal rhodopsin levels following an intense light exposure.

History The presenting symptom is nonprogressive impaired night vision, but given enough time to adapt in the dark, patients will achieve a normal sensitivity.

Epidemiology and Etiology The proposed defect in patients with FA appears to be an abnormal regeneration rate of the visual photoreceptor pigments.

GENETICS Autosomal recessive.

Clinical Signs

VISUAL ACUITY Usually unaffected.

FUNDUS Examination shows a multitude of yellow-white, tiny dots in the posterior pole that radiate out towards the periphery. The macula is almost invariably spared (Figure 6-17A–C).

Differential Diagnosis

Retinitis punctata albescens—this is a variant of retinitis pigmentosa in which the fundus shows yellow-white dots but has narrowed vessels and a severely reduced ERG that does not recover with dark adaptation.
Fleck retina of Kandori—a disorder with larger patch-like flecks and a less severe impairment of night vision.

Diagnostic Evaluation

VISUAL FIELDS Normal.

DARK ADAPTOMETRY Both the cone and rod components of the dark adaptation curve are very slow in reaching the final threshold.

ELECTRORETINOGRAPHY It is important to know that unless given enough time to dark adapt, both the a- and b-waves of the ERG are severely reduced. However, with prolonged dark adaptation, ERG returns to normal.

ELECTROOCULOGRAPHY There is slow recovery of the light rise with dark adaptation.

Prognosis and Management The defective night vision is nonprogressive, and the vision is usually unaffected.

Oguchi's Disease

Definition This variant of CSNB is characterized by a nonprogressive night vision impairment that is thought to be due to a defective phototransduction process.

Epidemiology and Etiology The visual photoreceptor pigments are normal, and the proposed defect is thought to be impaired phototransduction, giving rise to abnormal ERG findings.

Clinical Signs The retina has a peculiar silvery metallic sheen where retinal vessels stand out against the background fundus appearance. This unusual appearance may be seen in the entire retina or may be present only in the posterior pole or the periphery.

MIZUO–NAKAMURA PHENOMENON The retina has a metallic sheen following light adaptation, which disappears after few hours in the dark (Figure 6-18).

Diagnostic Evaluation

VISUAL FIELDS Normal.

DARK ADAPTOMETRY There is a normal cone adaptation but a markedly delayed rod adaptation that reaches a normal threshold level over a prolonged period of time (from 3 to 24 hours).

ELECTRORETINOGRAPHY Normal-amplitude a-wave and reduced or absent b-wave are seen under photopic and scotopic conditions. It is of note that even after the dark-adapted thresholds have returned to normal, the ERG b-wave may still be absent.

ELECTROOCULOGRAPHY Normal light rise.

Prognosis and Management The night vision defect is nonprogressive. There is no treatment available for Oguchi's disease.

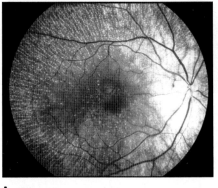

A

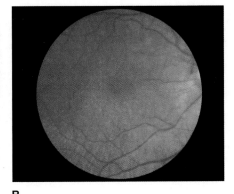

B

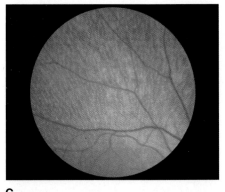

C

Figure 6-17 Fundus albipunctatus
*A. Red-free photograph showing radiating dots extending from the posterior pole to the retinal periphery. **B,C.** Multiple, yellow-white, tiny dots radiating out from the posterior pole toward the fundus periphery are visible in the color pictures. (Courtesy of Retina Slide Collection, Wills Eye Hospital, Philadelphia, Pennsylvania, compiled by Dr. Tamara Vrabec and Dr. Gordon Byrnes.)*

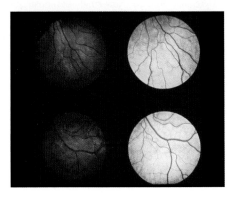

Figure 6-18 Mizuo-Nakamura phenomenon *Metallic sheen of the retina after light exposure* (right-hand photographs) *has disappeared after a few hours of dark adaptation* (left). *(Courtesy of Retina Slide Collection, Wills Eye Hospital, Philadelphia, Pennsylvania, compiled by Dr. Tamara Vrabec and Dr. Gordon Byrnes.)*

ALBINISM

Definition

Albinism is a group of conditions that involves the melanin system of the eye or skin, or both.

Classification

Ophthalmically, two clinical patterns are noted:

True albinism—congenitally subnormal vision and nystagmus are present.
Albinoidism—there is normal or minimally reduced vision and no nystagmus.

However, both clinical patterns share many clinical characteristics. True albinism is divided into the following two types:

Oculocutaneous albinism—both the eye and the skin are affected.
Ocular albinism—only the eyes appear to be affected.

Epidemiology and Etiology

Etiology Oculocutaneous albinism results from a reduction in the amount of primary melanin deposited in each melanosome, whereas ocular albinism is caused by a reduction in the total number of melanosomes.

Genetics

Oculocutaneous albinism—autosomal recessive
Ocular albinism—X-linked

Important Clinical Signs

Both ocular and oculocutaneous albinism share the following ocular clinical features:

Reduced visual acuity in the range of 20/40 to 20/400. The severity of visual deficit is proportional to the degree of fundus hypopigmentation (Figure 6-19).

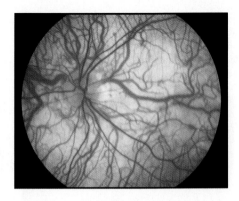

Figure 6-19 Albinism *Markedly hypopigmented fundus. Note the haphazard underlying large choroidal vessels. (Courtesy of Retina Slide Collection, Wills Eye Hospital, Philadelphia, Pennsylvania, compiled by Dr. Tamara Vrabec and Dr. Gordon Byrnes.)*

Nystagmus, light sensitivity, and a high degree of refractive errors.
Iris transillumination from decreased pigmentation.
Foveal aplasia or hypoplasia. In the presence of significant foveal hypoplasia, nystagmus begins within 2 to 3 months of life (Figure 6-20).
Hypopigmented retina from the periphery to the posterior pole.
Abnormal retinogeniculostriate projections where many temporal nerve fibers decussate rather than project to the ipsilateral geniculate body. This phenomenon accounts for the abnormal stereopsis in these patients.

The female carriers of ocular albinism may reveal partial iris transillumination and fundus hypopigmentation (Figure 6-21A,B).

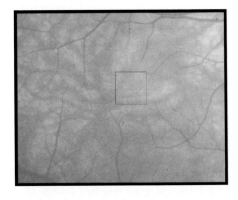

Figure 6-20 Albinism, foveal hypoplasia
Color fundus photograph concentrating on the foveal region of a patient with albinism. Note a complete absence of foveal architecture and foveal reflex—foveal hypoplasia (box). (Courtesy of Retina Slide Collection, Wills Eye Hospital, Philadelphia, Pennsylvania, compiled by Dr. Tamara Vrabec and Dr. Gordon Byrnes.)

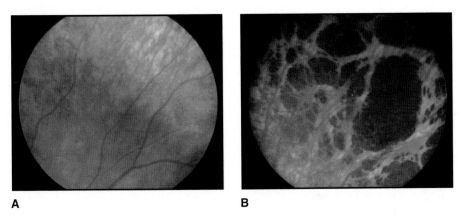

A   **B**

Figure 6-21 Albinism, female carrier *A,B. Partially hypopigmented fundus in a female carrier of ocular albinism. (Courtesy of Retina Slide Collection, Wills Eye Hospital, Philadelphia, Pennsylvania, compiled by Dr. Tamara Vrabec and Dr. Gordon Byrnes.)*

Associated Clinical Signs

Skin hypopigmentation is seen in patients with oculocutaneous albinism. Two forms of potentially lethal albinisms are observed:

Chédiak-Higashi syndrome—oculocutaneous albinism is combined with extreme susceptibility to infection that can often lead to death in childhood or youth.

Hermansky-Pudlak syndrome—oculocutaneous albinism with a platelet defect causing easy bruising and bleeding. Most patients with this disorder in the United States are of Puerto Rican origin.

Histology

Macromelanosomes in the eye or skin, or both

Increased number of decussating fibers at the chiasm

Diagnostic Evaluation

The typical constellation of symptoms and signs suggests the diagnosis. Asymmetric visually evoked cortical potentials occur due to abnormal decussation of the nerve fibers at the chiasm.

The tyrosinase hair bulb test indicates the presence or absence of the tyrosinase enzyme (it is required in the biosynthesis of melanin) and divides the oculocutaneous albinism into two types, tyrosinase-positive and tyrosinase-negative. Tyrosinase-negative albinos show a complete lack of pigmentation in the skin, hair, and eyes, whereas tyrosinase-positive albinos have some degree of pigmentation.

Hematologic consultation is necessary if Chédiak-Higashi or Hermansky-Pudlak syndromes are suspected (Figure 6-22).

Prognosis and Management

Because all forms of albinism are inherited, genetic counseling is important. A majority of children with albinism are able to attend regular schools with some degree of assistance, but only a few see well enough to drive. Refraction, tinted glasses, and visual aids are helpful for older patients. Hematologic consultation in an appropriate setting is mandatory.

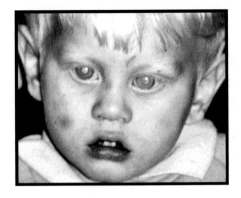

Figure 6-22   Oculocutaneous albinism, Hermansky-Pudlak Syndrome   *Purpuric patches on the cheeks, forehead, and left upper lid of a young boy with oculocutaneous albinism and Hermansky-Pudlak syndrome. (Courtesy of Retina Slide Collection, Wills Eye Hospital, Philadelphia, Pennsylvania, compiled by Dr. Tamara Vrabec and Dr. Gordon Byrnes.)*

RETINITIS PIGMENTOSA

Definition

Retinitis pigmentosa (RP) is a group of hereditary disorders associated with a primary abnormality of the photoreceptor-RPE complex, and is characterized subjectively by night blindness and a loss of peripheral vision, and objectively by a grossly reduced or extinguished full-field ERG. However, the hereditary basis can be established in only 50% of cases.

Epidemiology and Etiology

Onset   Variable and depends on the inheritance pattern.

Genetics   The following modes of inheritance have been described:

Sporadic—there is no family history of RP. These are the most common cases. Some of these cases are autosomal recessive, and others may represent autosomal-dominant mutations.

Autosomal dominant—next most common mode of inheritance and has the best prognosis.

Autosomal recessive.

X-linked recessive—least common group with worst prognosis.

History

Patients with typical RP present with a history of night blindness or nyctalopia (a complete or partially reduced rate of visual adaptation at night or in dim illumination). Patients may also have difficulty with peripheral vision in dim light. The difficulty with night vision may begin in early childhood, or patients may notice it in the second or third decade of life. By the age of 30 years, over 75% of patients are symptomatic.

Clinical Signs

Classic Clinical Triad   The classic clinical triad of RP includes (Figure 6-23):

1. Retinal "bone-spicule" pigmentation
2. Arteriolar attenuation
3. Waxy optic disc pallor (Figure 6-24A,B)

Additionally, vitreous debris is frequently encountered.

Important Clinical Signs   The following are the important clinical features of RP.

NIGHT BLINDNESS   The most common presenting clinical symptom. Peripheral vision problems are initially noticed only in the dim light, but later these problems are noted under all conditions. Eventually, only a small zone of central vision remains.

VISUAL ACUITY   The central vision may be preserved for many years in the autosomal-dominant form of RP. An early loss of central vision is often observed in the X-linked or autosomal-recessive forms. Additionally, cataract, cystoid macular edema, and surface wrinkling of the internal limiting membrane may contribute to early vision loss.

FUNDUS FINDINGS   Fundus findings may differ according to the stage of the disease.

Very early—arteriolar narrowing; fine dust-like intraretinal pigmentation.

Later features—perivascular "bone-spicule" pigment clumping. Pigmentary changes begin in the midretinal periphery and then extend anteriorly as well as posteriorly, giving rise to a ring scotoma. Waxy pallor of the optic disc is the least reliable sign of the RP triad.

Advanced features—unmasking of the large choroidal vessels, prominent arteriolar attenuation, and marked optic disc pallor.

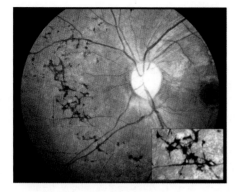

Figure 6-23   Retinitis pigmentosa (RP)
The classic clinical triad of waxy optic disc pallor, arteriolar attenuation, and "bone-spicule" pigmentation (inset) *in a patient with RP. (Courtesy of Retina Slide Collection, Wills Eye Hospital, Philadelphia, Pennsylvania, compiled by Dr. Tamara Vrabec and Dr. Gordon Byrnes.)*

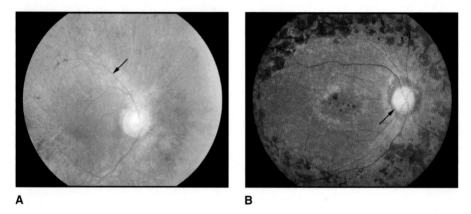

A   B

Figure 6-24   RP *Arteriolar attenuation (*inset, ***A**), optic disc pallor (*arrow, ***B**), and pigmentary changes in the fundus as are the characteristic findings in patients with RP. Visual acuity was reduced to finger counting vision due to foveal changes. (Courtesy of Retina Slide Collection, Wills Eye Hospital, Philadelphia, Pennsylvania, compiled by Dr. Tamara Vrabec and Dr. Gordon Byrnes.)*

MACULA Macular involvement may occur in the following ways:

Cystoid macular edema (may respond to systemic acetazolamide)
Surface wrinkling
Atrophic changes

Associated Ocular Features These features may include the following:

Optic nerve head drusen
Open-angle glaucoma (in 3% of patients with RP)
Posterior subcapsular cataract (common in all forms of RP)
Keratoconus
Myopia (frequently encountered)

Diagnostic Evaluation

A constellation of characteristic signs and symptoms helps establish the diagnosis.

Visual Fields Initially, there is a full or partial ring scotoma in the midperiphery, which extends anteriorly as well as posteriorly, leaving only a central island of vision in the late stages.

Dark Adaptometry An elevation of the rod as well as the cone segment of the dark adaptation curve occurs. Based on the dark adaptometry results, autosomal-dominant RP can be divided into two types:

Type I RP—early-onset nyctalopia with an early diffuse loss of the rod sensitivity relative to cone sensitivity
Type II RP—adult-onset nyctalopia with an equal loss of the rod and cone sensitivity

Electroretinography This may be significantly subnormal even when the fundus shows minimal changes. Severely reduced or almost extinguished scotopic ERG responses are observed, whereas the photopic ERG is relatively unaffected. The cone b-wave implicit times, as elicited by flicker stimuli, are almost always prolonged in all forms of electroretinography. The b-wave implicit time on the ERG may be prolonged in patients with predominant loss of rods rather than cones. Recently, distinctive ERG patterns in the type I and the type II autosomal-dominant forms of RP have been observed. The rod ERG is more severely affected than the cone ERG in type I RP, whereas rod and cone ERGs are equally abnormal in type II RP.

Electrooculography Almost invariably reduced.

Atypical Retinitis Pigmentosa

Retinitis punctata albescens—scattered white dots are located mostly between the posterior pole and equator.
Sector RP—only one or two quadrants of the fundus are involved (Figure 6-25).
Pericentric RP—pigmentary changes are confined to the area around the posterior pole.
Retinitis pigmentosa sine pigmento—pigmentary changes in the fundus are either minimal or absent.
Retinitis pigmentosa with exudative vasculopathy—Coats' disease-like appearance in the fundus.

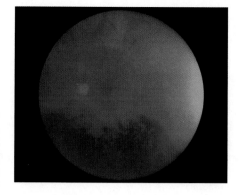

Figure 6-25   RP, sector variant *Equator-plus color fundus photograph showing inferior sectorial retinal pigmentary changes. (Courtesy of Retina Slide Collection, Wills Eye Hospital, Philadelphia, Pennsylvania, compiled by Dr. Tamara Vrabec and Dr. Gordon Byrnes.)*

Prognosis and Management

About one quarter of patients maintain good vision and are able to read throughout their lives. The autosomal-dominant form of the disease has the best prognosis, and the X-linked form has the worst prognosis. Only a few patients younger than 20 years of age will have a visual acuity of 20/400 or less. By age 50 years, however, a significant proportion of patients will have a visual acuity of approximately 20/400. Electroretinography is helpful in identifying the female carriers of X-linked RP (who may have a normal fundus), which may have implications for genetic counseling.

Appropriate investigations should be performed to rule out atypical forms of RP that may have an associated treatable systemic condition.

Explain to patients that not all people with RP go completely blind. Yearly followup is recommended to detect a precipitous fall in vision that may raise a possibility of a treatable cause, such as cystoid macular edema or cataract. Cystoid macular edema associated with RP responds favorably to oral acetazolamide, which is initially tried in a dose of 125 mg twice a day for 2 months to confirm its beneficial effect. If effective, acetazolamide may need to be continued for many months in some patients. Serial Goldmann perimetry should be performed at regular intervals to assess visual field changes. The role of oral vitamin A therapy in slowing the rate of progression of typical RP remains controversial. A variety of low-vision aids may be helpful.

SYSTEMIC DISEASES ASSOCIATED WITH RETINITIS PIGMENTOSA

Usher's Syndrome

Usher's syndrome is defined as congenital or progressive hearing loss associated with RP and is the most common syndrome associated with RP. Approximately 4% of children attending schools for the deaf have RP, and 50% of blind-deaf individuals have Usher's syndrome.

Pigmentary Retinopathy It is progressive and develops before puberty.

Systemic Features Usher's syndrome is divided into four subtypes, and types I and II constitute the majority of cases.

> *Type I*—profound congenital deafness, abnormal vestibular functions, and early-onset RP
> *Type II*—partial deafness, intact vestibular functions, and a milder form of RP

Bassen-Kornzweig Syndrome (Abetalipoproteinemia)

This disorder is thought to be caused by an inability of the body to synthesize apolipoprotein B, which helps in the absorption of fats in the small intestine.

Pigmentary Retinopathy It develops at the end of the first decade of life. Ptosis and ocular motility disturbances may also be seen.

Systemic Features Spinocerebellar ataxia, acanthocytosis, and abetalipoproteinemia are noted. Fat malabsorption and associated deficiency of fat-soluble vitamins, particularly A and E, is present, and jejunal biopsy is diagnostic.

Treatment Supplementation of vitamins A and E may be beneficial. Oral supplementation of vitamin A to reverse the psychophysical and electrophysiologic abnormalities remains controversial.

Refsum's Disease (Heredopathia Atactica Polyneuritiformis)

Refsum's disease is an autosomal-recessive disorder caused by a metabolic abnormality that results in a deposition of phytanic acid in many body tissues, including the eye.

Pigmentary Retinopathy Nyctalopia is almost always present. Fundus pigmentation is generally of a "salt-and-pepper" rather than "bone-spicule" type.

Systemic Features Hypertrophic peripheral neuropathy, cerebellar ataxia, deafness, ichthyosis, cardiac arrhythmias, and elevated cerebrospinal fluid protein.

Treatment Normalization of the elevated serum phytanic acid levels by a low phytanic acid diet may improve retinal function, and stop or slow the progression of disease.

Cockayne's Syndrome

Pigmentary Retinopathy "Salt-and-pepper type" with arteriolar attenuation and optic nerve pallor.

Systemic Features Childhood dwarfism with cachectic and prematurely aged appearance. Affected children have a small head with characteristic bird-like facies, and disproportionately large hands and feet. Deafness, photodermatitis, nystagmus, ataxia, and progressive mental retardation are associated features. Death may occur in the third or fourth decade of life.

Kearns-Sayre Syndrome

This syndrome is a mitochondrial myopathy in which an increased number of distorted mitochondria are accumulated in the skeletal muscles (including the extraocular muscles), retinal pigment epithelium, and heart. Histologically, affected muscles show "ragged-red" fibers, caused by the accumulation of mitochondria beneath the plasma membrane and between myofibrils.

Pigmentary Retinopathy Variable appearance. Diffuse retinal pigment epithelial mottling may be observed.

Systemic Features Combination of chronic progressive external ophthalmoplegia (most common finding), pigmentary retinopathy, and complete heart block (may cause death). This condition usually becomes manifest before the age of 20 years.

Bardet-Biedl Syndrome

Pigmentary Retinopathy "Bull's-eye" maculopathy occurs in most cases. A few cases are similar to typical RP with "bone-spicule" pigmentation.

Systemic Features Mental handicap, polydactyly, obesity, and hypogenitalism; renal abnormalities (in most cases).

Laurence-Moon Syndrome

Retinopathy Either typical RP type or choroidal atrophy.

Systemic Features Spastic paraplegia, mental handicap, and hypogenitalism.

Mucopolysaccharidoses

This group of metabolic disorders is caused by a deficiency of lysosomal enzymes involved in the degradation of many mucopolysaccharides, such as dermatan sulphate, heparan sulphate, and keratan sulphate. An abnormal deposition of the nondegraded mucopolysaccharides leads to multiple organ system dysfunction.

Genetics Autosomal recessive, except Hunter's disease, which is X-linked recessive.

Ocular Features Retinal pigmentary degeneration—found in Hurler's, Hunter's, and Sanfilippo's diseases; corneal stromal infiltration; optic nerve head swelling; optic atrophy; and glaucoma (rare).

Systemic Features Facial coarseness, skeletal anomalies, and heart disease.

Neuronal Ceroid Lipofuscinosis (Batten Disease)

This group of disorders is characterized by an accumulation of autofluorescent lipopigments in the neurons as well as in nonneural tissues.

Types   Four types are differentiated, as follows:

INFANTILE TYPE (HAGBERG-SANTAVUORI)

Generalized retinal degeneration
Brownish discoloration of the macula
Early visual loss
Optic atrophy
Mental retardation and motor abnormalities between the ages of 1 and $1^1/_2$ years

LATE INFANTILE TYPE (JANSKY-BIELSCHOWSKY)

Generalized retinal degeneration and optic atrophy
Seizures and psychomotor problems with an onset between 2 and 4 years of age

JUVENILE TYPE (SPIELMEYER-VOGT)

Most common
"Bull's-eye" maculopathy with eventual development of RP-like clinical picture—may need to be differentiated from Stargardt's disease
Reduced vision
Progressive mental deterioration
Seizures (occasionally)
Average age of death—17 years

ADULT-ONSET (KUFS)

No ocular abnormalities
Benign; not fatal

Friedreich's Ataxia

Friedreich's ataxia is an autosomal-recessive inherited disorder caused by a disturbance of pyruvate metabolism. Onset of symptoms is noted between 10 and 20 years of age.

Ocular Features

Pigmentary retinopathy
Vestibular nystagmus
Optic atrophy
Vertical gaze paresis

Systemic Features

Cerebellar ataxia
Absence of tendon reflexes
Scoliosis
Cardiomyopathy—often the cause of death in the third to fourth decade of life

CARCINOMA-ASSOCIATED RETINOPATHY SYNDROME

Definition

Carcinoma-associated retinopathy (CAR) syndrome is a visual paraneoplastic disorder in which autoantibodies against tumor antigen cross-react with retinal proteins, resulting in rod and cone photoreceptor dysfunction.

Synonym—paraneoplastic retinopathy.

Epidemiology and Etiology

Age   Variable.

Sex   No preference.

Etiology   Associated malignancies are:

Small cell carcinoma of the lung (most common)
Gynecologic, breast, endocrine, or other visceral malignancies

In CAR syndrome, autoantibodies cross-react with the protein recoverin, located within the photoreceptors.

History

The typical presentation is severe, progressive, bilateral visual loss over a period of months, with relatively unremarkable fundus. Visual symptoms may precede diagnosis of the underlying malignancy.

Clinical Signs

Cone Dysfunction   As evidenced by:

Decreased visual acuity
Photosensitivity
Reduced color vision
Central scotoma

Rod Dysfunction   As evidenced by:

Nyctalopia
Prolonged dark adaptation
Ring scotoma

Fundus Features

Early stages—may be normal
(Figure 6-26A–D)
Late findings—narrow retinal arterioles
Retinal pigment epithelial mottling
Optic nerve pallor

Associated Clinical Features

Systemic features of the underlying malignancy may or may not be present.

Differential Diagnosis

Decreased vision from retinal cause and normal-appearing fundus
Stargardt's disease
Cone dystrophy
Twig branch retinal vein occlusion
Twig branch retinal artery occlusion
Toxic retinopathy
Reperfused central retinal artery occlusion

Age, family and medication history, bilaterality, fluorescein angiography, and the electrophysiologic tests help to differentiate CAR syndrome from the preceding disorders.

Diagnostic Evaluation

Typical set of symptoms and signs
Color vision—reduced
Visual fields—typically, ring scotoma
Dark adaptometry—prolonged dark adaptation
Electroretinography—reduced amplitudes of both rod and cone responses
Serum anti-recoverin antibodies
Systemic oncologic evaluation

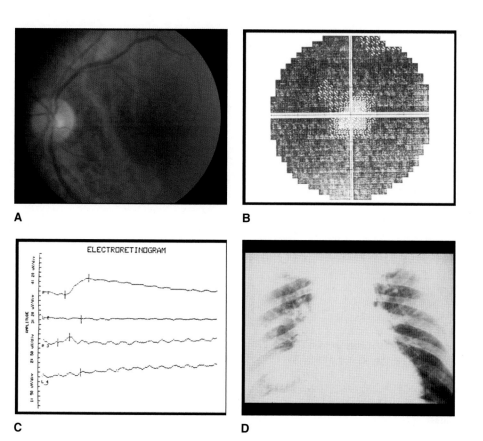

Figure 6-26   Carcinoma-associated retinopathy (CAR) syndrome   *A. Normal fundus but decreased vision. **B**. Severe and generalized visual field depression. **C**. Near completely extinguished electroretinogram. **D**. Mass lesion in the right lower lobe of the lung diagnosed as small cell carcinoma causing CAR syndrome. (Courtesy of Dr. William Tasman and the Retina Slide Collection, Wills Eye Hospital, Philadelphia, Pennsylvania, compiled by Dr. Tamara Vrabec and Dr. Gordon Byrnes.)*

Prognosis and Management

If photoreceptors are sufficiently damaged, visual functions are usually permanently altered. Various treatment measures have been tried, but their role in improving the visual prognosis remains to be proven. These measures include treatment of the underlying malignancy, steroids, plasmapheresis, and intravenous immunoglobulins.

Chapter 7

RETINAL AND CHOROIDAL TUMORS

Franco M. Recchia, MD

ASTROCYTIC HAMARTOMA

Definition

Astrocytic hamartoma is a congenital, minimally progressive, benign tumor arising from the glial cells of the retina and usually located around the optic disc. It is often associated with the systemic condition tuberous sclerosis (Bourneville's disease), occasionally with neurofibromatosis, but also occurs sporadically in otherwise normal individuals.

Epidemiology and Etiology

Most astrocytic hamartomas occur congenitally in association with tuberous sclerosis (TS), a familial phakomatosis characterized by the triad of seizures, mental retardation, and skin lesions. TS has an estimated incidence of 1 in 15,000 to 1 in 100,000 and exhibits autosomal-dominant inheritance. Roughly one half of patients with TS possess astrocytic hamartomas. Causative genes have been identified on chromosomes 9q34 and 16p13.

History

Patients with astrocytic hamartomas are usually asymptomatic. Visual field testing may reveal a scotoma in the area corresponding to the tumor.

Important Clinical Signs

The appearance of a retinal astrocytic hamartoma is principally of two types:

1. Smaller, noncalcified, flat, smooth tumor that appears as mild thickening of the nerve fiber layer
2. Larger, calcified, whitish-yellow nodular mass ("mulberry lesion")

Aspects of both may be seen in the same lesion, as it is likely that calcification progresses slowly over many years (Figure 7-1).

Every patient with an astrocytic hamartoma of the retina or optic nerve *must* be evaluated for TS. Typical manifestations of TS include:

Skin lesions (~95% incidence)—(1) Hypomelanotic macules: oval ("ash-leaf"), polygonal, or punctate ("confetti") in shape. Usually present at birth and often the first presenting sign. (2) Reddish-brown papular rash over the face (termed *adenoma sebaceum,* but actually angiofibromas), often mistaken for acne. Rarely present before a few years of age.

Seizures (~90% incidence)—myoclonic spasms lasting 10 to 50 seconds; tend to become *grand mal* type later in life.

Mental retardation (~60% incidence).

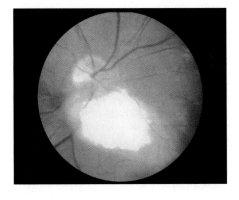

Figure 7-1 Astrocytic hamartoma

A peripapillary astrocytic hamartoma can be seen with classic mulberry calcification overlying an underlying smooth tumor. Patients and family members should be examined for tuberous sclerosis. (Courtesy of Drs. Jerry and Carol Shields, Oncology Service, Wills Eye Hospital, Philadelphia, Pennsylvania.)

Associated Clinical Signs

Ocular Occasionally, may produce vitreous hemorrhage, vitreous seeding, subretinal hemorrhage, or retinal detachment.

Systemic (Additional manifestations of TS.) Ungual fibromas, pleural cysts (leading to spontaneous pneumothorax), renal angiomyolipoma, cardiac rhabdomyoma, and hamartomas of the liver, thyroid, pancreas, or testis may occur.

Differential Diagnosis

Retinoblastoma
Myelinated nerve fibers
Retinal granuloma
Drusen of the optic disc
Papillitis

Diagnostic Evaluation

Fluorescein Angiography The tumor appears relatively hypofluorescent in the arterial phase.

Superficial fine blood vessels are seen during the venous phase. The tumor stains intensely and homogeneously in the late phases.

B-scan Ultrasonography A larger, calcified lesion often appears as a discrete, oval, solid mass with a sharp anterior border.

Neuroimaging Subependymal hamartomas characteristic of TS may be seen with computed tomography (CT) or magnetic resonance imaging (MRI).

Prognosis and Management

The vast majority of retinal astrocytic hamartomas are asymptomatic and do not require treatment. Associated retinal detachment can often be treated with demarcating laser photocoagulation. Patients and family members should be examined regularly for manifestations of TS.

RETINOBLASTOMA

Definition

Retinoblastoma is the most common intraocular malignancy of children. It may be familial but most often is sporadic in occurrence. The tumor arises from cells in the developing retina of one or both eyes as a result of mutations in the retinoblastoma (Rb) tumor-suppressor gene. Retinoblastoma presents most often as a white intraocular mass with propensity for direct extension into the brain and almost certain mortality if untreated.

Epidemiology and Etiology

This tumor occurs in approximately 1 in 15,000 live births. Most children are diagnosed at a mean of 18 months. No predilection for race or gender has been shown. Roughly two thirds of cases are unilateral, and one third are bilateral. Unilateral cases are more likely to be diagnosed at an older age (mean of 24 months) and are most often nonfamilial (sporadic). Bilateral cases are diagnosed at a mean of 12 months, are usually familial, and are nearly always multifocal.

The tumor results from mutations or loss of both alleles of the Rb gene, located on chromosome 13q14. The Rb gene product appears to function as regulator of cellular proliferation through inhibitory effects on gene transcription at specific stages of the cell cycle. The timing of allelic inactivation determines whether the mutation is *germinal* (i.e., heritable by offspring of the affected child) or *somatic* (nonheritable). In germinal cases, a mutant allele is present before fertilization, most commonly as a result of inheritance from either parent. In somatic cases, both alleles are present and active at fertilization, and spontaneous mutations in each allele arise subsequently.

History

A white pupillary reflex (leukokoria; Figure 7-2) and strabismus are the two most common findings reported by parents. In fewer than 10% of cases is a family history known at the time of diagnosis.

Important Clinical Signs

Most patients present with leukokoria and strabismus. Small retinoblastomas appear as flat, translucent, white retinal lesions (Figure 7-3A). With growth, the tumor appears more solid, elevated, and chalky-white, with overlying dilated tortuous blood vessels.

Three growth patterns have been described: (1) endophytic, in which the tumor grows from the retina inward to seed the vitreous cavity or anterior chamber; (2) exophytic, in which the tumor grows from the retina outward to occupy the subretinal space, often causing an exudative retinal detachment (Figure 7-3B); and (3) diffuse infiltrating, the least common form, characterized by shallow spread of tumor along the entire retina and into the vitreous and anterior chamber.

Other important findings are iris neovascularization, which occurs in nearly one fifth of all cases, and "pseudohypopyon" (settling of tumor and inflammatory cells in the anterior chamber).

Associated Clinical Signs

Clear lens
Heterochromia iridis
Spontaneous hyphema
Extrascleral extension
Pinealoblastoma ("trilateral retinoblastoma")

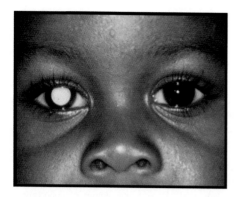

Figure 7-2 Retinoblastoma *This young boy has leukokoria and strabismus, the most common clinical presentation of retinoblastoma. (Courtesy of Drs. Jerry and Carol Shields, Oncology Service, Wills Eye Hospital, Philadelphia, Pennsylvania.)*

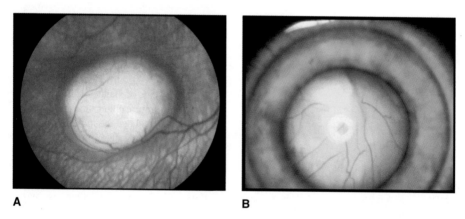

A B

Figure 7-3 Retinoblastoma *A. Focal retinoblastoma presenting as a macular intraretinal amelanotic tumor. B. Massive exophytic retinoblastoma with tumor behind the clear lens. (Courtesy of Drs. Jerry and Carol Shields, Oncology Service, Wills Eye Hospital, Philadelphia, Pennsylvania.)*

Differential Diagnosis

Leukokoria

Coats' disease
Persistent fetal vasculature syndrome (formerly termed *persistent hyperplastic primary vitreous,* or PHPV)
Toxocariasis
Retinopathy of prematurity
Familial exudative vitreoretinopathy
Retinal astrocytoma
Cataract
Norrie's disease
Incontinentia pigmenti

Vitreous Seeding

Intraocular inflammation
Endophthalmitis
Vitreous hemorrhage
Leukemic infiltration

Diagnostic Evaluation

Examination Detailed systemic evaluation and examination is required, as well as family history and ocular examination of parents, and complete examination of both eyes (often requiring anesthesia for complete visualization of the fundi with scleral depression).

Ultrasonography An elevated, rounded, intraocular mass is seen, with high internal reflectivity (calcification) and shadowing of sclera and soft tissue posterior to the lesion.

Computed Tomography A CT scan is helpful in detecting intraocular calcification (present in roughly 80% of retinoblastomas), assessing extraocular extension, and identifying the presence of pineal tumors.

Fluorescein Angiography The angiogram reveals early arterial filling of the vessel feeding the tumor, leakage of dye from intrinsic tumor vessels, and late hyperfluorescence of the tumor.

Prognosis

Spontaneous regression is rare and leads to phthisis bulbi. Typically, if untreated, children die within 2 years of diagnosis. Early detection, coupled with improvements and promptness of treatment, has reduced the mortality rate to less than 10%. The main determinant for mortality is optic nerve invasion. For this reason, it is imperative to obtain as long a section of optic nerve as possible during enucleation.

Prognostic factors for failure to preserve vision or to preserve the eye are larger tumor size, vitreous seeding, and macular involvement.

Children with germinal retinoblastoma have an increased risk of developing other primary malignancies over the course of their lifetimes. These tumors include principally intracranial retinoblastoma, osteogenic sarcoma of the long bones, and sarcoma of soft tissues. The risk is estimated to be 20% within 25 years of treatment.

Management

Children diagnosed with retinoblastoma should undergo evaluation for systemic involvement, including complete blood count, lumbar puncture, neuroimaging, and bone marrow biopsy. Genetic testing of the child and family members should be performed.

Individual treatment varies according to number, size, and location of tumors, as well as systemic status. Therapeutic options include cryotherapy, laser photocoagulation, enucleation, external beam irradiation, plaque radiotherapy, chemotherapy, thermotherapy, and chemothermotherapy.

Chemoreduction prior to definitive ocular treatment may be helpful in reducing the need for enucleation and reducing the rate of occurrence of pinealoblastoma.

In familial cases, genetic counseling provides parents with important information regarding the probability of further occurrences. Patients with germinal retinoblastoma must be warned of the possibility of transmission to their offspring.

RETINAL CAPILLARY HEMANGIOMA

Definition

Originally termed *angiomatosis retinae,* retinal capillary hemangioma is a benign vascular tumor of variable size located in the retina or adjacent to optic disc. Usually diagnosed by the fourth decade, it may be the first manifestation of von Hippel-Lindau (VHL) disease, a familial cancer syndrome with which it is commonly associated.

Epidemiology and Etiology

This tumor may occur in a sporadic or hereditary fashion. Retinal capillary hemangioma occurs in up to 80% of patients with VHL syndrome and is often the first manifestation, diagnosed at a mean age of 25 years. The VHL syndrome has an estimated prevalence of 1 in 40,000 and is possibly more common in whites. It exhibits dominant inheritance and has variable phenotypes within families. Mean survival of patients with VHL is 41 years of age.

Von Hippel-Lindau syndrome is caused by mutations in the VHL gene, a tumor-suppressor gene located on chromosome 3p25. The function of the VHL gene is unknown but is speculated to regulate the expression and function of hypoxia-responsive angiogenic factors (e.g., vascular endothelial growth factor [VEGF]).

History

Capillary hemangiomas may be diagnosed incidentally or in patients suspected of having VHL syndrome. The tumors may be asymptomatic or may produce painless visual impairment from vitreous hemorrhage, macular pucker, or retinal detachment.

Important Clinical Signs

Retinal Capillary Hemangioma Usually located peripherally and well circumscribed. Initially appears as a yellow-red dot with a min-imally dilated "feeding" arteriole or draining venule (Figure 7-4). With growth, appears orange-red with more prominently dilated afferent and efferent vessels. May have associated exudation, subretinal fluid, or preretinal fibrosis.

Juxtapapillary Capillary Hemangioma Orange-red in color, but less well circumscribed. It often lacks feeder vessels.

Von Hippel-Lindau Syndrome Hemangioblastomas of the cerebellum and spinal cord, renal cell carcinoma, or pheochromocytoma.

Associated Clinical Signs

Retinal detachment and, rarely, neovascular glaucoma may complicate capillary hemangioma. Hemangiomas of the adrenal glands, lungs, and liver, and multiple cysts of the pancreas and kidneys, have been observed in some patients with VHL syndrome.

Differential Diagnosis

Retinal Capillary Hemangioma

Other tumors—retinal cavernous hemangioma, racemose hemangioma, choroidal melanoma, and astrocytic hamartoma

Vascular diseases—Coats' disease, retinal arterial macroaneurysm, familial exudative vitreoretinopathy, and exudative macular degeneration

N.B.: A distinction has been made between the retinal angioma of VHL syndrome and an acquired, nonhereditary entity occurring in older patients and termed *vasoproliferative retinal tumor*. This latter condition is usually located in the inferotemporal peripheral fundus and lacks markedly dilated feeder vessels.

Optic Disc Hemangioma

Papillitis
Optic disc granuloma
Optic disc glioma

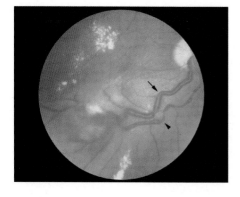

Figure 7-4   Retinal capillary hemangioma   *Note the dilated feeding retinal arteriole* (arrow) *and the segmented draining retinal vein* (arrowhead) *with associated macular edema, premacular fibrosis, and lipid exudation. These lesions may be the first manifestation of von Hippel-Lindau disease. (Courtesy of Drs. Jerry and Carol Shields, Oncology Service, Wills Eye Hospital, Philadelphia, Pennsylvania.)*

Diagnostic Evaluation

Ocular   Fluorescein angiography is the most helpful ancillary study. In the arterial phase, a prominent, dilated feeder arteriole may be seen. The tumor appears hyperfluorescent early and remains so through the late phases, sometimes leaking dye into the vitreous. Ultrasonography may be helpful in diagnosing lesions of greater than 1 mm and demonstrates acoustic solidity throughout the lesion.

Systemic   All patients with retinal capillary hemangioma, as well as relatives, should be evaluated for VHL syndrome. Genetic testing for mutations in the VHL gene is available.

Prognosis and Management

The natural history is variable, with both progressive enlargement and spontaneous regression having been reported. Visual prognosis is highly variable and depends on tumor location, size, and associated complications, especially those that involve the macula. In patients with VHL syndrome, risk of developing associated tumors increases with age. Morbidity and mortality are related to these associated tumors. Median survival is less than 50 years, with renal carcinoma as the leading cause of death.

Treatment is recommended for tumors with documented growth or effects on visual function. The goal of treatment is to induce resolution of exudation or subretinal fluid. Laser photocoagulation is reserved for smaller tumors (less than 2 mm in diameter). Larger tumors are best treated with cryotherapy or plaque radiotherapy. Vitreoretinal surgery, and, rarely, enucleation may be necessary for patients with advanced or uncontrollable pathology.

Patients with VHL syndrome and their relatives should be examined regularly for life. This includes regular testing for urine catecholamines, CT and ultrasonography of the kidneys, and MRI of the brain.

RETINAL CAVERNOUS HEMANGIOMA

Definition

Retinal cavernous hemangioma is a benign, rarely progressive, vascular tumor of the retina or optic disc characterized by a collection of venous aneurysms. It may be associated with similar vascular anomalies of the skin and central nervous system.

Epidemiology and Etiology

Tumor occurrence is mostly sporadic. Small pedigrees of patients with cavernous hemangioma as part of a dominantly inherited oculoneurocutaneous syndrome have been reported.

History

Patients are usually asymptomatic, but the tumor may produce painless visual loss. A hereditary component may be noted.

Important Clinical Signs

A cluster of dark-red, intraretinal aneurysms is located along a retinal venule, appearing as a "cluster of grapes" arising from the inner retinal surface (Figure 7-5). Often there is overlying gray fibroglial tissue. Usually the tumor does *not* have associated exudation or a feeding arteriole.

Associated Clinical Signs

Vitreous hemorrhage occurs in up to 10% of cases. There may also be cutaneous vascular malformations. Cavernous hemangiomas of the midbrain or cerebellum may produce seizures or subarachnoid hemorrhage.

Differential Diagnosis

Capillary hemangioma
Acquired vasoproliferative tumor
Racemose hemangioma
Coats' disease

Diagnostic Evaluation

Fluorescein angiography produces a typical pattern: the lesion is hypofluorescent in the early arterial phase and exhibits slow hyperfluorescence during the late venous phase as dye enters the venous channels. A fluorescein-blood interface may be seen within the aneurysms in the late phases of the angiogram.

Prognosis and Management

Most cavernous hemangiomas do not enlarge and can be managed with periodic observation. The main complication is vitreous hemorrhage, although this rarely causes permanent visual loss. Tumors causing recurrent vitreous hemorrhage may be treated with cryotherapy, laser photocoagulation, or plaque radiotherapy.

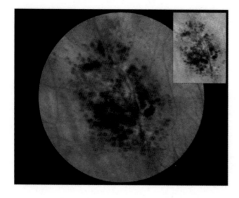

Figure 7-5 Retinal cavernous hemangioma *Note the "cluster of grapes" appearance of these intraretinal aneurysms* (inset). *There is a lack of exudation, and surface grey retinal fibrous tissue is noted. (Courtesy of Drs. Jerry and Carol Shields, Oncology Service, Wills Eye Hospital, Philadelphia, Pennsylvania.)*

CONGENITAL HYPERTROPHY OF THE RETINAL PIGMENT EPITHELIUM

Definition

Congenital hypertrophy of the retinal pigment epithelium (CHRPE) is a benign, asymptomatic condition, consisting of one or more well-demarcated, pigmented, flat, nonprogressive lesions, usually found in the equatorial or peripheral fundus. In rare instances, multifocal lesions may be associated with familial colonic polyposis.

Epidemiology and Etiology

The condition is probably congenital. It occurs with equal frequency in blacks and whites.

History

Patients are usually asymptomatic. Often the disorder is noted as an incidental finding during ophthalmoscopy.

Important Clinical Signs

Two forms have been described:

Solitary—unilateral, deeply pigmented, flat, circular lesion measuring 1 to 6 mm in diameter. Usually sharply demarcated, the lesion may be solid black, or ringed with a small border of hypopigmentation. Lacunar areas of depigmentation within the lesion may be seen (Figure 7-6A).

Multifocal—also termed *congenital grouped pigmentation* or "bear tracks." Groups of 3 to 30 small (0.1 to 2 mm) lesions typically appear in one sector of the midperipheral retina. Usually they lack the internal lacunae and hypopigmented halo of the solitary form.

Multifocal fundus lesions resembling CHRPE have been reported in close association with Gardner's syndrome (Figure 7-6B,C), a familial condition of colonic polyps and extraintestinal osteomas and fibromas with invariable progression to colonic cancer. The lesions associated with Gardner's syndrome, however, are bilateral, have irregular borders, and are often scattered in the fundus.

Differential Diagnosis

Malignant choroidal melanoma
Choroidal nevus
Combined hamartoma of the retina and retinal pigment epithelium (RPE)

Diagnostic Evaluation

Diagnosis is based on typical ophthalmoscopic features. By fluorescein angiography, the tumor exhibits persistent hypofluorescence. Lacunar areas are seen as hyperfluorescent, consistent with depigmentation of the RPE.

Prognosis and Management

Most CHRPE lesions are nonprogressive and require only periodic examination. In rare instances, mild enlargement may occur. Patients with bilateral lesions suggestive of those seen in Gardner's syndrome should be referred for colonoscopy.

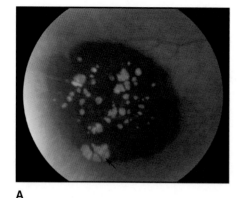

A

Figure 7-6A   Congenital hypertrophy of the retinal pigment epithelium *Note the sharp, discrete borders of the lesion as well as the lacunar areas of depigmentation* (arrow) *within the lesion. (Courtesy of Drs. Jerry and Carol Shields, Oncology Service, Wills Eye Hospital, Philadelphia, Pennsylvania.)*

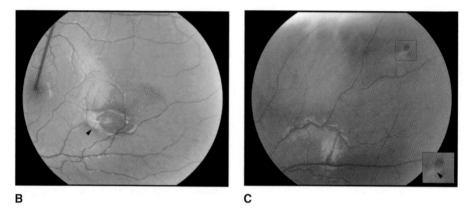

B   **C**

Figure 7-6B,C   Pigmented fundus lesion, Gardner's syndrome *Pigmented lesion associated with Gardner's syndrome and familial gastrointestinal cancer. A depigmented "tail"* (arrowheads) *is noted adjacent to the pigmented fundus lesion (**B, C** inset). (Courtesy of Drs. Jerry and Carol Shields, Oncology Service, Wills Eye Hospital, Philadelphia, Pennsylvania.)*

COMBINED HAMARTOMA OF THE RETINA AND RETINAL PIGMENT EPITHELIUM

Definition

Combined hamartoma of the retina and RPE is a benign, slightly elevated, partially pigmented tumor located around the optic nerve or in the peripheral fundus. It is composed histologically of proliferated glial cells, fibrovascular tissue, and pigment epithelial cells.

Epidemiology and Etiology

The tumor is often diagnosed by early adulthood. The preponderance of cases in infants and young children suggests that the lesion may be congenital. An association of combined hamartomas, usually macular and sometimes bilateral, has been seen with neurofibromatosis (most commonly type 2).

History

In cases of juxtafoveal lesions, there is painless visual loss from epimacular membrane traction or subretinal exudation.

Important Clinical Signs

Juxtapapillary Variant Ill-defined, elevated, charcoal-grey mass adjacent to, or overlying, the optic disc. A grey-white membrane overlying the tumor causes stretching of retinal blood vessels and retinal striae, often involving the macula (Figure 7-7).

Peripheral Variant Slightly elevated, pigmented ridge concentric to the optic disc. There is dragging of dilated retinal vessels toward the lesion by the overlying membrane.

Associated Clinical Signs

Choroidal neovascularization
Vitreous hemorrhage
Manifestations of neurofibromatosis type 2 (bilateral acoustic neuromas, brain meningiomas, spinal cord schwannomas, posterior subcapsular cataracts)

Differential Diagnosis

Choroidal melanoma
Choroidal nevus
Reactive hyperplasia of the RPE
Melanocytoma
When lightly pigmented and occurring in children, may be mistaken for retinoblastoma or toxocariasis

Diagnostic Evaluation

Diagnosis is based on ophthalmoscopic features. Fluorescein angiography reveals multiple, dilated, fine blood vessels within the tumor, which may become hyperfluorescent as the angiogram progresses.

Prognosis and Management

Because lesions are usually not progressive, regular observation is appropriate. However, contraction of overlying fibroglial tissue leads to macular distortion, secondary retinoschisis, and retinal holes. In cases of visual loss, vitrectomy and membrane stripping may be performed, but visual recovery is limited.

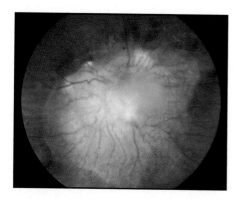

Figure 7-7 Combined hamartoma of the retina and retinal pigment epithelium
This is an example of the juxtapapillary variant of the lesion. The edge of an apparent membrane is noted most prominently on the nasal aspect of the lesion. There is marked distortion and tortuosity of the involved retinal vasculature. (Courtesy of Drs. Jerry and Carol Shields, Oncology Service, Wills Eye Hospital, Philadelphia, Pennsylvania.)

CHOROIDAL NEVUS

Definition

Choroidal nevus is a common, benign tumor of the posterior fundus. Although usually flat or minimally elevated, and grey or brown in appearance, it may show variable degrees of pigmentation.

Epidemiology

Prevalence in the general population is estimated to be 1% to 6%. The tumor occurs much more commonly in whites.

History

Patients are usually asymptomatic, and the tumor is generally discovered incidentally during routine ophthalmoscopy. Vision may be reduced from extension of associated subretinal fluid into the macula, or from an associated serous retinal detachment.

Important Clinical Signs

The tumor is most often slate-grey or brown in color, but it may be heterogeneously pigmented or even amelanotic (pale yellow). Choroidal nevi are usually 1 to 5 mm in diameter, flat or minimally elevated (less than 2 mm in anteroposterior dimension), with ill-defined margins. Drusen overlying the tumor are common and signify chronicity of the lesion (Figure 7-8). Alterations of the overlying RPE include pigment clumping and fibrous metaplasia (yellow-white plaques). "Orange pigment" at the level of the RPE represents aggregates of macrophages containing lipofuscin granules and may suggest growth or malignant transformation of the nevus.

Associated Clinical Signs

Serous detachment of the neurosensory retina or RPE
Choroidal neovascularization

Differential Diagnosis

Pigmented Lesion

Choroidal melanoma
Congenital hypertrophy of the RPE
Combined hamartoma of the retina and RPE
Subretinal hemorrhage

Amelanotic Lesion

Circumscribed choroidal hemangioma
Choroidal osteoma
Choroidal metastasis
Inflammatory lesion

Diagnostic Evaluation

Diagnosis is based on characteristic ophthalmoscopic features. Fluorescein angiography, although not specific for choroidal nevus, may provide confirmatory evidence. Areas of deep pigmentation are hypofluorescent, whereas areas of overlying RPE alteration will appear hyperfluorescent. Ultrasonography may be helpful for establishing baseline thickness.

Prognosis and Management

All small choroidal melanocytic tumors have the potential for malignant transformation and metastasis. Risk factors for growth include greater thickness (larger than 1 mm), proximity to the optic disc, orange pigment on the surface of the tumor, and presence of subretinal fluid. The chance of growth of small, flat ("nonsuspicious") lesions lacking these clinical features is less than 5%.

Management consists of baseline photographs and regular examination to establish quiescence or growth of the nevus. Serial photographs, ultrasonography, and more frequent examinations are indicated in cases of suspected growth.

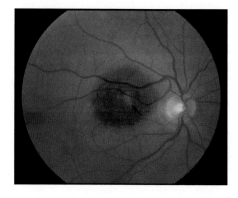

Figure 7-8   Choroidal nevus   *This is a minimally elevated choroidal pigmented lesion with overlying drusen* (arrow). *No orange pigment or submacular fluid suggestive of potential transformation of a malignant choroidal melanoma is noted. (Courtesy of Drs. Jerry and Carol Shields, Oncology Service, Wills Eye Hospital, Philadelphia, Pennsylvania.)*

CHOROIDAL MELANOMA

Definition

Choroidal melanoma is the most common primary intraocular malignancy, occurring most often in white adults. Dome-shaped or mushroom-shaped, this variably pigmented mass arises from the choroid of one eye. It has a propensity for metastasis to the liver.

Epidemiology and Etiology

The incidence is 1 in 2000 to 1 in 2500 in Caucasians. In the United States, choroidal melanoma is nearly ten times more common in whites than in African Americans. There is no gender predilection. The tumor is uncommon in people younger than 30, but incidence increases with age and the average age at diagnosis is in the sixth decade.

Risk factors may include prolonged exposure to ultraviolet light, congenital oculodermal melanocytosis (nevus of Ota), and family history. The tumor arises from dendritic melanocytes of the choroid. There are two major categories of cells histopathologically: spindle cells and epithelioid cells. Rare associated karyotypic abnormalities have been reported, most commonly alterations of chromosome 6.

History

The malignancy is usually asymptomatic and painless. Visual effects include blurred vision, floaters, photopsia, and visual field defects.

Important Clinical Signs

The tumor appears as a dome-shaped, elevated choroidal mass, typically confined to the subretinal space. About 20% of choroidal melanomas will break through Bruch's membrane and take on a characteristic mushroom shape. Color varies from brown to grey to pale-yellow (amelanotic), with overlying clumps of orange pigment, representing collections of lipofuscin

(Figure 7-9A,B). Associated subretinal fluid, usually surrounding the base of the lesion, may be noted, and the tumor may lead to total serous retinal detachment.

Associated Clinical Signs

Vitreous hemorrhage
Subretinal hemorrhage
Choroidal neovascularization
Extrascleral extension with orbital invasion

Differential Diagnosis

Choroidal nevus
Choroidal metastasis
Combined hamartoma of the retina and retinal pigment epithelium
Congenital hypertrophy of the RPE (CHRPE)
Circumscribed choroidal hemangioma, reactive hyperplasia of the RPE
Bilateral diffuse uveal melanocytic proliferation
Choroidal osteoma

Diagnostic Evaluation

Diagnosis is based on ophthalmoscopic features. Ultrasonography reveals an acoustically hollow, dome-shaped or mushroom-shaped mass with low internal reflectivity. Ultrasonographic measurements of tumor thickness are valuable in determination of doses for radiotherapy, as well as for serial evaluation following treatment.

Fluorescein angiography of small choroidal tumors shows early mottled hyperfluorescence of the tumor with progressive staining in the late phases. Large tumors display filling of large intrinsic vessels in the venous phase, with diffuse late staining.

Prognosis

Overall, 5-year survival for patients with choroidal melanoma is about 80%. Median

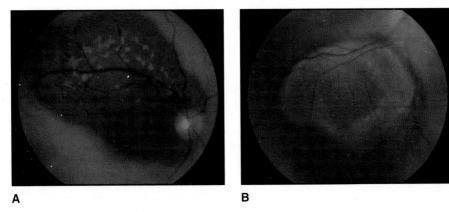

A

B

Figure 7-9   Choroidal melanoma   *A. A large, elevated, pigmented choroidal mass surrounding the temporal aspect of the optic disc is appreciated with overlying orange pigment. The primary goal of treatment of choroidal melanoma is prevention of systemic metastases. B. A large, elevated, pigmented choroidal mass with subretinal fluid and orange pigment. Orange pigment may represent macrophage ingestion of lipofuscin pigment and reflect tumor activity. (Courtesy of Drs. Jerry and Carol Shields, Oncology Service, Wills Eye Hospital, Philadelphia, Pennsylvania.)*

survival is about 7 years. Prognosis for survival depends on a variety of factors, including age at diagnosis, intraocular location, extent of metastasis, tumor size, and tumor cell type. The 5-year mortality for patients with epithelioid melanomas is 42%; for those with spindle cell tumors, 10%. The 5-year mortality for patients with tumors with largest basal tumor diameter (LTD) greater than 15 mm is nearly 50%; for those with LTD less than 10 mm, under 20%.

Risk factors for metastasis include documented growth, proximity to the optic disc, and greater tumor thickness. Nearly one half of patients with metastatic choroidal melanoma die within 1 year of treatment. There appears to be no difference in mortality in patients treated initially with enucleation when compared with those treated with iodine-125 plaque radiotherapy.

Management

Ocular   The primary goal of treatment of choroidal melanoma is prevention of metastasis. Choice of specific modality depends on tumor size, location, and the patient's systemic and psychological status.

Enucleation remains the standard treatment for large melanomas (greater than 12 mm in LTD and 8 mm in thickness). Other options for smaller tumors include: transpupillary thermotherapy (TTT), radiotherapy (plaque brachytherapy or proton-beam irradiation), and local resection (reserved for anterior lesions). Observation is appropriate for small tumors with little evidence of growth.

Patients should be evaluated regularly with careful funduscopy, serial fundus photographs, and ultrasonography.

Systemic   The vast majority (~98%) of patients have no discernible metastasis at the time of diagnosis of their choroidal melanoma. Baseline systemic evaluation should be performed in every patient, under the direction of a medical oncologist. Assessment typically includes complete blood count, liver enzyme panel, chest roentgenogram, and imaging (i.e., CT or ultrasound) of the abdomen. Measurement of liver enzymes should be performed regularly along with ophthalmoscopy.

CHOROIDAL MELANOCYTOMA

Definition

Choroidal melanocytoma is a benign, minimally progressive, deeply pigmented tumor occurring at or around the optic nerve. It is probably a variant of choroidal nevus.

Epidemiology

Blacks and whites are affected equally. Malignant melanomas, by contrast, occur much less frequently in black patients.

History

Patients are usually asymptomatic. Visual loss may occur in rare instances of tumor growth or retinal vascular obstruction. No inheritance pattern has been recognized.

Important Clinical Signs

Characteristically, this charcoal-grey or grey-black tumor is located on or adjacent to the optic disc, with both a deep choroidal component and superficial extension into the nerve fiber layer (Figure 7-10). It is usually unilateral. A relative afferent papillary defect (RAPD) may be seen in up to 30% of cases.

Associated Clinical Signs

The uninvolved area of the optic disc may become acutely edematous with an associated decline in vision. Rarely, neovascular glaucoma secondary to vascular obstruction may occur.

Differential Diagnosis

Juxtapapillary choroidal melanoma
Choroidal nevus
Hyperplasia of the RPE
Combined hamartoma of the retina and RPE

Diagnostic Evaluation

Diagnosis is based on characteristic ophthalmoscopic features. Regular examinations and serial fundus photographs are essential for documentation of growth or malignant transformation.

Prognosis and Management

The patient is followed by observation. Roughly 15% of melanocytomas will exhibit small degrees of enlargement. However, malignant transformation is possible and is often heralded by more rapid growth and visual changes. In such cases, enucleation of the affected eye should be considered.

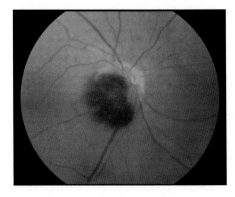

Figure 7-10   Choroidal melanocytoma
Note the dark brown lesion involving the optic disc. There are feathery edges to the lesion. A small percentage (~15%) of melanocytomas will demonstrate some growth; malignant transformation is rare but has been reported. (Courtesy of Drs. Jerry and Carol Shields, Oncology Service, Wills Eye Hospital, Philadelphia, Pennsylvania.)

CHOROIDAL METASTASIS

Definition

Choroidal metastasis is the most common intraocular malignancy, visible ophthalmoscopically in up to 1% of patients with systemic malignancy (most commonly arising from the lung or breast). Clinically it is apparent as an amelanotic, shallow, round or oval choroidal mass posterior to the equator. Choroidal metastasis is usually unilateral but may be multifocal and bilateral. It is the presenting sign of metastatic malignancy in up to one third of patients.

Epidemiology and Etiology

There is a cumulative lifetime incidence of 1 in 400 to 1 in 1000 Americans. At autopsy, microscopic intraocular lesions are detectable in 5% to 10% of patients with systemic malignancy; of these, 10% have clinically apparent lesions. The increasing incidence is likely attributable to increased survival of patients with cancer, improved detection, and greater awareness.

The most common primary malignancy is breast carcinoma in women and lung carcinoma in men. In patients with no known primary site at the time of diagnosis, systemic evaluation leads to diagnosis of lung carcinoma in one third of patients and breast carcinoma in one tenth of patients. Known primary sites other than breast and lung comprise less than 10% of cases with choroidal metastasis. In one half of patients, however, a primary site is not discovered.

Tumors are overwhelmingly carcinomas, rarely sarcomas. Spread is hematogenous. Cytologic findings are consistent with the tumor of origin.

History

Blurred vision (usually painless) is reported in 80% of patients. Floaters and visual field defects are other symptoms, along with eye pain (5% to 15%). A history of malignancy is noted in 65% to 75% of patients.

Important Clinical Signs

The tumor appears as a round or oval, placoid, minimally elevated choroidal mass that is variable in color. It is unifocal and unilateral in roughly two thirds of cases. Metastases from breast and lung are typically pale-yellow, whereas those from cutaneous melanoma are dark grey or brown (Figure 7-11A,B). Other tumors with characteristic coloration include metastatic renal cell and thyroid carcinoma (typically orange-red) and metastatic carcinoid tumors (typically pink or yellow-orange). Typically the tumor is located posterior to the equator (greater than 90%); it is predominantly macular in roughly 10%. Tumor growth may result in disc edema and serous retinal detachment.

Associated Clinical Signs

Conjunctival injection
Hyperopic shift
Neovascular glaucoma

Differential Diagnosis

Amelanotic choroidal melanoma
Circumscribed choroidal hemangioma
Retinal astrocytoma
Choroidal osteoma
Intraocular lymphoma
Sclerochoroidal calcification
Central serous chorioretinopathy
Choroidal granuloma
Posterior scleritis
Vitelliform dystrophy

Diagnostic Evaluation

Fluorescein angiography of carcinoma metastatic to the choroid shows early hypofluorescence of the lesion with a relative paucity of intrinsic vessels, and diffuse hyperfluorescence of the tumor in the late phases of the study. Indocyanine green

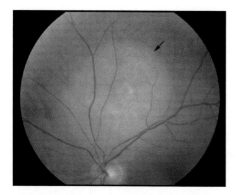

Figure 7-11A Choroidal metastasis
Metastatic lung cancer presents as an amelanotic choroidal lesion (arrow) *superior to the optic disc. Most choroidal metastases occur posterior to the equator. They may be unifocal or multifocal. (Courtesy of Drs. Jerry and Carol Shields, Oncology Service, Wills Eye Hospital, Philadelphia, Pennsylvania.)*

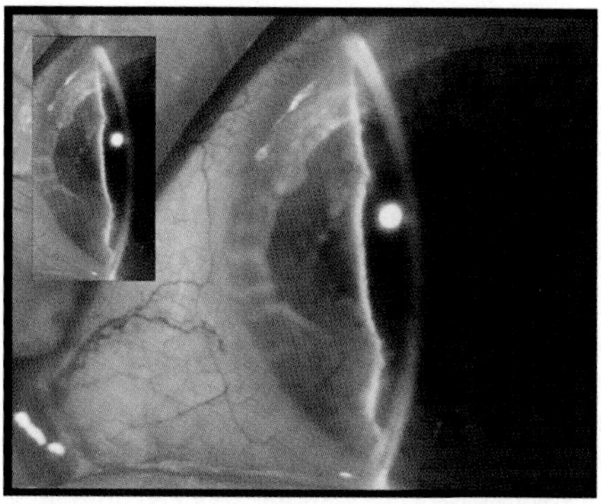

Figure 7-11B Choroidal metastasis to iris *Metastatic breast cancer presents initially to the patient as an amelanotic iris mass.*

angiography may demonstrate additional, smaller choroidal tumors.

Ultrasonography is most helpful for elevated tumors; they appear hyperechoic (bright) with high internal reflectivity. Fine-needle aspiration biopsy may be helpful, especially in patients with no known malignancy.

Prognosis

Most metastatic tumors are relentlessly progressive and tend to grow faster than primary choroidal malignancies. If untreated, bullous retinal detachment can lead to blindness and secondary angle-closure glaucoma.

Optic disc edema causes profound and often irreversible visual loss. Factors related to the preservation of vision and eye structures include number and size of tumors, proximity to the optic nerve and fovea, and responsiveness to therapy.

Survival is related to effective treatment and remission of systemic disease. Patients with

choroidal metastasis from breast carcinoma tend to survive longer than patients with choroidal metastases from other sites.

Management

Ocular Choroidal metastases are most often treated with external-beam radiotherapy, chemotherapy, hormonal therapy, or a combination. Single, smaller tumors may be treated effectively with plaque radiotherapy.

Systemic Patients with systemic disease should be referred to a medical oncologist. Management of patients with a known primary extraocular malignancy requires a staging evaluation appropriate for the primary tumor. Patients with no known primary site at time of diagnosis are evaluated with a thorough physical examination (with attention to breasts and lymph nodes), mammography, chest roentgenogram, CT of the chest and abdomen, and bone scan.

CHOROIDAL HEMANGIOMA

Definition

Choroidal hemangioma is a benign vascular tumor that occurs in two forms: circumscribed (discrete) and diffuse. The circumscribed variant is a well-defined, orange-red, dome-shaped mass, usually occurring in the posterior fundus and diagnosed by the fourth decade of life. The diffuse variant is characteristically associated with Sturge-Weber syndrome (encephalotrigeminal angiomatosis) and is diagnosed at a younger age. It gives a markedly asymmetric, bright red reflex to the fundus of the involved eye.

Epidemiology

Circumscribed Type Sporadic, usually diagnosed in third or fourth decade. May be worsened by pregnancy. Usually unilateral.

Diffuse Type Diagnosed in childhood. Occurs in roughly one-third of patients with Sturge-Weber syndrome. Usually unilateral and ipsilateral to the characteristic facial hemangioma (nevus flammeus, or "port-wine stain"), but may be bilateral and associated with bilateral facial hemangiomas.

History

Patients may be asymptomatic. Visual impairment is usually painless and results from hyperopic shift (in cases of submacular tumor) or subretinal fluid.

Important Clinical Signs

Circumscribed Type

Discrete, slightly elevated, orange-red mass arising in the posterior choroid

Serous retinal detachment in two thirds of cases

Overlying RPE metaplasia or retinoschisis (Figure 7-12)

Diffuse Type

Bright red color involving a large section (more than 50%) of the fundus

Tortuosity of overlying retinal vessels

Shifting subretinal fluid

Manifestations of Sturge-Weber syndrome include facial nevus flammeus (100% of patients), cerebral abnormalities, and intracranial calcifications. Asymmetric cupping of the optic nerve (due to congenital glaucoma) occurs, particularly in cases of nevus flammeus involving the ipsilateral upper eyelid.

Associated Clinical Signs

Choroidal neovascularization (circumscribed type)

Retinitis pigmentosa-like changes (diffuse type)

Differential Diagnosis

Central serous retinopathy

Amelanotic choroidal melanoma

Choroidal metastasis

Choroidal inflammation

Diagnostic Evaluation

Fluorescein angiography and indocyanine green angiography reveal early hyperfluorescence corresponding to filling of choroidal vessels feeding the tumor. B-scan ultrasonography demonstrates a dome-shaped elevation in the case of a circumscribed hemangioma and marked choroidal thickening in cases of diffuse tumors.

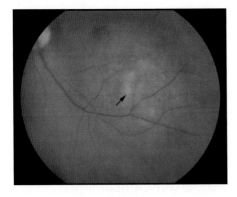

Figure 7-12   Choroidal hemangioma, circumscribed type *A macular choroidal hemangioma demonstrates submacular fluid and overlying retinal pigment epithelial metaplasia* (arrow). *This lesion is often confused with central serous retinopathy. (Courtesy of Drs. Jerry and Carol Shields, Oncology Service, Wills Eye Hospital, Philadelphia, Pennsylvania.)*

Prognosis and Management

Management consists of observation as long as patients are asymptomatic. In cases of macular involvement or extensive retinal detachment, visual impairment is inevitable, and treatment is indicated.

Treatment consists of radiation therapy (external beam, cobalt-60 brachytherapy, or proton-beam irradiation). Delimiting laser photocoagulation, external drainage, or scleral buckling is indicated for retinal detachment.

INTRAOCULAR LYMPHOMA

Definition

Intraocular lymphoma is a malignant, indolent, often bilateral, lymphocytic proliferation with diffuse infiltration of the posterior segment that occurs in two forms: (1) arising primarily from the eye or central nervous system (CNS); or (2) systemic, usually visceral, lymphoma, metastatic to the uvea. Most often it affects older patients and is associated with CNS lymphoma. Intraocular lymphoma was formerly termed *reticulum cell sarcoma*.

Epidemiology and Etiology

Usually this lymphoma affects immunocompetent patients in their sixth to seventh decade. It is bilateral in up to 90% of cases. A more aggressive form is seen in patients who are severely immunocompromised, most commonly from the acquired immunodeficiency syndrome (AIDS). Intraocular lymphoma is the presenting sign of CNS lymphoma in 80% of patients, but may precede CNS involvement by up to 10 years (mean of 2 years). The incidence appears to be increasing, possibly as a result of more widespread immunosuppression or improved diagnosis.

Most often the lymphoma is a large-cell B lymphocytic (i.e., non-Hodgkin) tumor. It is thought to arise from cells of the retina, RPE, brain, meninges, and spinal cord.

History

Patients have a history of floaters and painless visual loss. Chronic, unremitting vitritis that is unresponsive to corticosteroids occurs, along with neurologic impairment.

Important Clinical Signs

Vitreous inflammation
Multiple, yellow-white lesions deep to the retina that progressively enlarge and coalesce
Overlying pigmentary alterations

Associated Clinical Signs

Anterior uveitis
Retinal vasculitis, leading to vascular obstruction (Figure 7-13)
Optic disc edema

Differential Diagnosis

Vitritis

Amyloidosis
Old vitreous hemorrhage
Senile vitritis

Retinal Infiltrates and Vasculitis

Toxoplasmosis
Cytomegalovirus retinitis
Acute retinal necrosis
Sarcoidosis

Subretinal Infiltrates

Multifocal choroiditis
Acute posterior multifocal placoid pigment epitheliopathy
Multiple evanescent white dot syndrome
Fundus flavimaculatus
Choroidal granuloma
Amelanotic choroidal melanoma
Choroidal metastasis
Bilateral diffuse uveal melanocytic proliferation

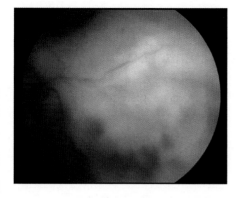

Figure 7-13   Intraocular lymphoma
Hazy photograph demonstrating vitritis and intraretinal invasion of lymphoma with associated hemorrhagic retinal vasculitis. (Courtesy of Drs. Jerry and Carol Shields, Oncology Service, Wills Eye Hospital, Philadelphia, Pennsylvania.)

Diagnostic Evaluation

In the absence of known CNS disease, vitreous biopsy (through either fine-needle aspiration or pars plana vitrectomy) has the greatest diagnostic yield. Multiple vitreous specimens may be needed.

Prognosis and Management

All patients with intraocular lymphoma should be evaluated for CNS and systemic involvement, by neurologic examination, neuroimaging (thin-section magnetic resonance imaging), lumbar puncture, and bone marrow biopsy. Untreated, most patients die within a few years of diagnosis. Patients with disease limited to the eye may be treated with external beam irradiation only. Adjunct chemotherapy and corticosteroids prolong survival to a median of 41 months (with 22% disease-free at 5 years), but do not decrease the risk of subsequent CNS involvement. Ocular relapse, especially within the first year after treatment, is common.

CHOROIDAL OSTEOMA

Definition

Choroidal osteoma is a rare, benign choroidal tumor composed of mature bone, occurring most commonly in the posterior pole of one eye of healthy young women.

Epidemiology and Etiology

The tumor most often affects women younger than 30 years of age. It is unilateral in 75% of cases and usually sporadic, but rare familial cases have been reported.

History

Patients are usually asymptomatic. Diminished visual acuity or metamorphopsia are caused by macular involvement by the tumor.

Important Clinical Signs

The tumor is most often adjacent to, or surrounding, the optic disc. It appears pale-yellow to orange in color and is minimally elevated (usually less than 2 mm in thickness). Overlying clumping of brown, grey, or orange pigment may be noted (Figure 7-14).

Associated Clinical Signs

Choroidal neovascularization
Serous retinal detachment

Differential Diagnosis

Amelanotic choroidal melanoma
Carcinoma metastatic to the choroid
Circumscribed choroidal hemangioma
Disciform scar of age-related macular degeneration
Idiopathic sclerochoroidal calcification

Diagnostic Evaluation

Diagnosis is based on typical ophthalmoscopic features. Fluorescein angiography reveals early mottled hyperfluorescence and late diffuse staining. Leakage from associated choroidal neovascularization may be seen. B-scan ultrasonography demonstrates a mildly elevated, highly reflective choroidal mass with acoustic shadowing. Computed tomography reveals focal hyperintensity similar to bone in the affected choroid.

Prognosis and Management

Prognosis is variable. Visual loss may result from degeneration of the overlying RPE, choroidal neovascularization, or retinal detachment. Management consists of observation and, as appropriate, laser photocoagulation to choroidal neovascularization.

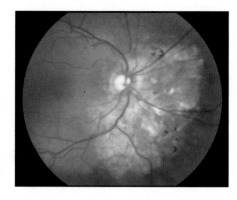

Figure 7-14   Choroidal osteoma
Peripapillary choroidal osteoma is yellow-white in color and there are some overlying areas of clumping of brown pigment. B-scan ultrasonography of choroidal osteoma shows a highly reflective choroidal mass with acoustic shadowing behind the lesion; this is due to intrinsic bone. (Courtesy of Drs. Jerry and Carol Shields, Oncology Service, Wills Eye Hospital, Philadelphia, Pennsylvania.)

Chapter 8

CONGENITAL AND PEDIATRIC RETINAL DISEASES

J. Arch McNamara, MD

RETINOPATHY OF PREMATURITY

Definition

Retinopathy of prematurity (ROP) is a proliferative retinopathy of premature, low-birth-weight infants.

Epidemiology and Etiology

Infants born at less than 36 weeks' gestation or those with a birth weight of 2000 g or less who have received oxygen therapy are at risk. Examinations should start at 6 weeks after birth. Infants who are born weighing 1000 g or less are at particularly high risk of developing severe ROP.

The retinal vasculature of infants born prematurely has not completed its growth to the anterior extent of the retina. The developing vasculature is susceptible to capillary endothelial cytotoxicity. Preexisting vessels are damaged and neovascularization develops off the surface of the retina. Continued growth and contraction of fibrovascular tissue may lead to retinal detachment.

History

Infants at high risk for ROP should be screened for characteristic findings.

Important Clinical Signs

The posterior segment signs of ROP follow a progression of increasing severity that were classified according to the International Classification of ROP (ICROP). First the location of the disease is determined, then the stage of severity, and finally the extent of that stage is noted (Table 8-1, Figures 8-1 through 8-5).

Associated Clinical Signs

"Plus" disease denotes increased severity. When an eye has dilation and tortuosity of the retinal vessels in the posterior pole, then it is said to have plus disease and has a poorer prognosis (Figure 8-6). When vascularization is only present in zone I and there is plus disease, then a very poor prognosis exists because of the risk of rapid progression ("rush" disease).

"Threshold" disease is a level of ROP at which it is predicted that there is a 50% chance of progression to retinal detachment without treatment. It is characterized by 5 contiguous clock hours of extraretinal fibrovascular proliferation with plus disease or 8 accumulated clock hours of extraretinal fibrovascular proliferation (ERFP) with plus disease (Figure 8-7). When threshold disease is reached, treatment is recommended.

TABLE 8-1 INTERNATIONAL CLASSIFICATION OF RETINOPATHY OF PREMATURITY (ICROP)

Location

Zone I	Posterior circle of retina centered on the optic nerve with a radius of twice the disc-fovea distance
Zone II	Circular area of retina from the edge of zone I to the nasal ora serrata
Zone III	Remaining temporal crescent of retina

Extent

Number of clock hours or 30-degree sectors involved

Severity

Stage 1	Demarcation line between posterior vascularized retina and anterior avascular retina
Stage 2	Demarcation line with height, width, and volume (ridge)
Stage 3	Ridge with extraretinal fibrovascular proliferation (ERFP); may be mild, moderate, or severe
Stage 4	Subtotal retinal detachment
4A	Extrafoveal
4B	Involving the fovea
Stage 5	Total retinal detachment; always funnel-shaped
	Open anteriorly, open posteriorly
	Open anteriorly, narrow posteriorly
	Narrow anteriorly, open posteriorly
	Narrow anteriorly, narrow posteriorly

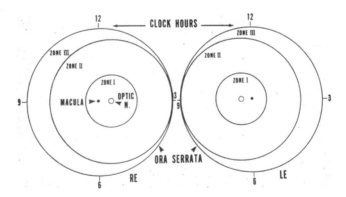

Figure 8-1 Retinopathy of prematurity (ROP) *Schematic diagram of division of fundus into zones for defining location of involvement with ROP.*

Occasionally neovascular tissue may form buds of vascular proliferation behind the ridge or demarcation line. These lesions are called "popcorn" because of their similarity to popped corn (see Figure 8-3A). These lesions do not carry any prognostic significance unless they are a part of ERFP at the advancing border of vascularization. Vitreous hemorrhage and preretinal hemorrhage can occasionally be seen in eyes with severe ERFP.

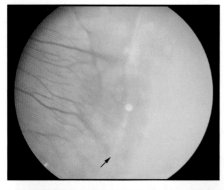

Figure 8-2   ROP, stage 2   *The demarcation line* (arrow) *between posterior vascularized and anterior avascular retina is elevated as a ridge.*

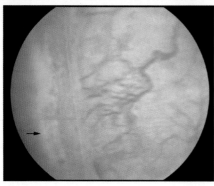

A

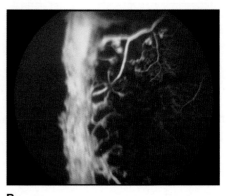

B

Figure 8-3   ROP, stage 3   *A. The ridge has fibrovascular tissue and is elevated off the surface of the retina (extraretinal fibrovascular proliferation, or ERFP). This is an example of severe stage 3 ROP. Buds of vascular proliferation behind the ridge are "popcorn" lesions* (arrow). *B. Fluorescein angiogram from same patient as in (A) showing intense hyperfluorescence from vascular proliferative tissue in region of ridge.*

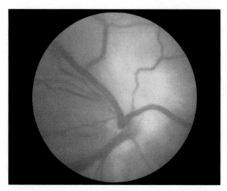

Figure 8-4   ROP, stage 5   *Eye with shallow total retinal detachment. Note loss of choroidal detail due to shallow subretinal fluid accumulation in posterior pole.*

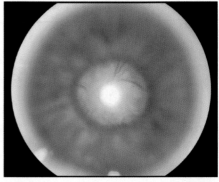

Figure 8-5   ROP, stage 5   *This eye has a total tractional retinal detachment due to severe fibrous proliferation with contraction of the fibrous tissue. Note the vascularized tissue behind the clear lens.*

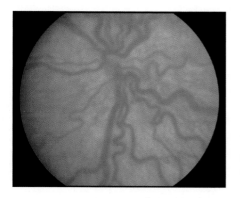

Figure 8-6   ROP, plus disease   *Dilation and tortuosity of vessels in the posterior pole denotes progressive disease and is known as "plus" disease.*

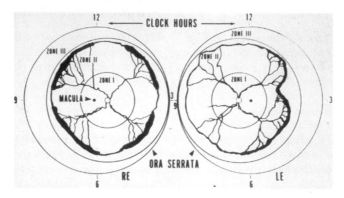

Figure 8-7   ROP, threshold disease   *Schematic diagram of threshold disease according to the Cryotherapy for Retinopathy of Prematurity Study Group. (Reprinted by permission of American Medical Association from Cryotherapy for Retinopathy of Prematurity Cooperative Group. Multicenter trial of cryotherapy of retinopathy of prematurity: Preliminary results. Arch Ophthalmol 1988; 106:474.)*

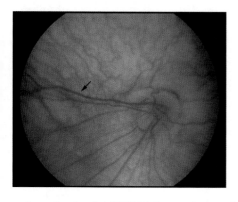

Figure 8-8   ROP   *Severe dragging of the temporal retina with vascular straightening* (arrow) *is a late cicatricial complication of ROP. Compare with familial exudative vitreoretinopathy, in* **Figure 8-18A.**

In early cicatricial ROP (after resolution of the acute phase) there may be a variety of tractional complications. A hallmark finding of regressed cicatricial ROP is temporal retinal dragging (Figure 8-8). After regression of ROP, either spontaneously or with treatment, several associated abnormalities may occur (Table 8-2).

TABLE 8-2   LATE COMPLICATIONS OF RETINOPATHY OF PREMATURITY

Myopia
Astigmatism
Strabismus
Amblyopia
Cataract
Glaucoma
Macular ectopia
Retinal fold
Retinal detachment—rhegmatogenous or exudative

Differential Diagnosis

The clinical setting usually aids in the diagnosis of ROP. Infants are born prematurely and are of low birth weight with a history of oxygen exposure.

Differential diagnosis depends on the stage of the disease. In less severe ROP, conditions that cause peripheral retinal vascular changes and retinal dragging should be considered (Table 8-3). In advanced cicatricial ROP, the differential diagnosis is that of retinal detachment or a white pupillary reflex, or both (Table 8-4).

Diagnostic Evaluation

Careful examination of neonates with indirect ophthalmoscopy in the intensive care nursery or at discharge commencing at 6 weeks of age is essential to detect ROP at a stage where treatment can be applied.

Prognosis and Management

The majority of infants who develop ROP undergo spontaneous regression (85%). However, 7% of infants weighing less than 1251 g at birth will develop threshold ROP.

Cryotherapy to the anterior avascular zone (Figure 8-9A,B) has been shown to reduce the likelihood of an unfavorable outcome (retinal fold through zone I, retinal detachment, or retrolental fibroplasia) by 50% in the Cryotherapy for ROP Study. Visual results are commensurately improved.

Laser photocoagulation delivered with an indirect ophthalmoscope to the anterior avascular zone has virtually replaced cryotherapy for threshold ROP (Figure 8-10A,B). Better visual outcomes have been achieved with laser treatment.

More advanced stages of ROP (stages 4 and 5 retinal detachment) can be treated with scleral buckling or vitrectomy, or both. The prognosis for visual recovery after retinal detachment remains poor.

TABLE 8-3   DIFFERENTIAL DIAGNOSIS OF EARLY STAGES OF RETINOPATHY OF PREMATURITY

Familial exudative vitreoretinopathy (FEVR)
Incontinentia pigmenti (Bloch-Sulzberger syndrome)
X-linked retinoschisis
Norrie's disease

TABLE 8-4 DIFFERENTIAL DIAGNOSIS OF LATE STAGES OF RETINOPATHY OF PREMATURITY

Cataract
Familial exudative vitreoretinopathy (FEVR)
Persistent fetal vasculature (PFV)
Ocular toxocariasis
Intermediate uveitis
Coats' disease
Retinoblastoma
Vitreous hemorrhage
Retinal detachment
Endophthalmitis

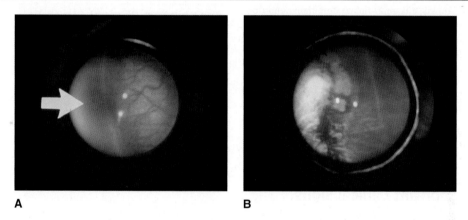

A   **B**

Figure 8-9   ROP, cryotherapy   *A. The* arrow *points to the anterior avascular zone where cryotherapy will be placed for threshold ROP.* ***B.*** *Late postoperative appearance of cryotherapy. Note regression of extraretinal fibrovascular proliferation.*

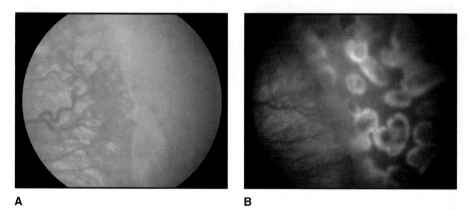

A   **B**

Figure 8-10   ROP   *A. Preoperative appearance of an eye with posterior threshold ROP.* ***B.*** *Late postoperative appearance after laser photocoagulation. Note regression of extraretinal fibrovascular proliferation.*

INCONTINENTIA PIGMENTI

Definition

Incontinentia pigmenti, or Bloch-Sulzberger syndrome, is a rare X-linked dominant condition that includes ocular, skin, central nervous system, skeletal, and other systemic abnormalities.

Epidemiology and Etiology

The pathogenesis of incontinentia pigmenti is unknown. It is an X-linked dominant condition that is usually lethal in males and thus usually only seen in female infants. However, an affected male with Klinefelter syndrome (xxy) or a genetic mosaicism may survive.

History

Characteristic skin changes usually start days after birth, with ophthalmic findings developing in infancy or even later in life.

Important Clinical Signs

Approximately one third of infants with incontinentia pigmenti have ocular findings. Fundus abnormalities include dilated, tortuous retinal vessels, peripheral retinal capillary nonperfusion with arteriovenous anastomoses and neovascularization (Figures 8-11 and 8-12), foveal hypoplasia, branch artery occlusions, neovascularization of the disc, retinal dragging, tractional and rhegmatogenous retinal detachments, retinal folds, vitreous hemorrhage, and optic disc pallor. The ocular abnormalities are often extremely asymmetric.

Associated Clinical Signs

Other ocular findings include cataract, conjunctival pigmentation, and strabismus. Skin findings, for which the disease is named, include vesicular skin eruptions (Figure 8-13) that later turn into depigmented lesions (Figure 8-14). These changes start days after birth.

Dental abnormalities consisting of missing or cone-shaped teeth are present in approximately two thirds of affected individuals (Figure 8-15). Associated central nervous system abnormalities include seizures, spastic paralysis, and mental retardation.

Differential Diagnosis

See Table 8-3, earlier. If retinal detachment is a presenting finding, other causes of infantile retinal detachment should be considered.

Diagnostic Evaluation

Clinical evaluation including examination of the skin may lead to a diagnosis of incontinentia pigmenti.

Prognosis and Management

Most patients with incontinentia pigmenti require no treatment. Progressive peripheral retinal neovascularization may respond to laser photocoagulation or cryotherapy. Retinal detachments may be repaired with scleral buckling or vitrectomy, or both.

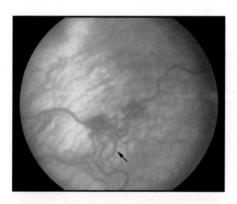

Figure 8-11   Incontinentia pigmenti
Peripheral fundus of a patient with incontinentia pigmenti showing peripheral retinal capillary nonperfusion and arteriovenous anastomoses (arrow).

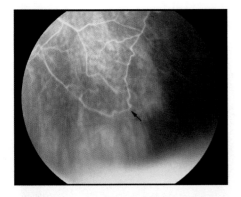

Figure 8-12   Incontinentia pigmenti
Fluorescein angiogram of the peripheral fundus of a patient with incontinentia pigmenti showing peripheral retinal capillary nonperfusion and arteriovenous anastomoses (arrow).

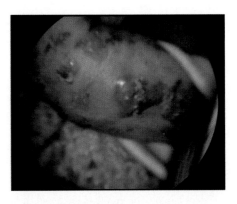

Figure 8-13   Incontinentia pigmenti, dermatologic findings   *Vesicular skin lesions in an infant with incontinentia pigmenti.*

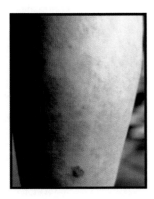

Figure 8-14   Incontinentia pigmenti, dermatologic findings   *Pigmentary alteration of the skin in a patient with resolved vesicular eruptions of incontinentia pigmenti.*

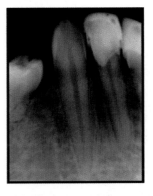

Figure 8-15   Incontinentia pigmenti, dental findings   *Dental x-ray of cone-shaped tooth in a patient with incontinentia pigmenti.*

FAMILIAL EXUDATIVE VITREORETINOPATHY

Definition

Familial exudative vitreoretinopathy (FEVR) is an autosomal-dominant fundus disorder characterized by peripheral retinal nonperfusion and neovascularization.

Epidemiology and Etiology

The exact etiology of FEVR is unknown. It is an autosomal-dominant hereditary disorder (rare cases of X-linked inheritance have been reported) that is asymptomatic in 50% of cases.

History

Infants born with FEVR are otherwise healthy. There is usually no history of prematurity, oxygen exposure, or respiratory difficulties. The clinical features vary considerably and, although bilateral, there is often asymmetry. Infants may present with strabismus or a white pupillary reflex if the findings are severe. However, symptoms of decreased vision may occur at any age.

Important Clinical Signs

The classic finding in FEVR is peripheral retinal capillary nonperfusion (Figure 8-16). Peripheral neovascularization may form at the border of posterior vascularized and anterior avascular retina (Figure 8-17A,B). Retinal dragging from contraction of fibrovascular tissue may occur (Figure 8-18A,B). Vitreous hemorrhage rarely occurs. Progression to more severe changes such as tractional, exudative, and even rhegmatogenous retinal detachment may occur (Figure 8-19). Intraretinal and subretinal lipid exudation may sometimes occur. The findings are often asymmetric.

Associated Clinical Signs

In severe cases with retinal detachment, there may be cataract, band keratopathy, neovascular

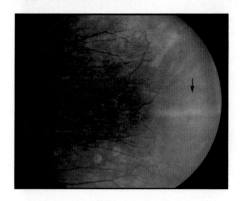

Figure 8-16   Familial exudative vitreoretinopathy (FEVR) *Peripheral retinal capillary nonperfusion* (arrow) *in FEVR appears featureless.*

glaucoma, phthisis, or a combination of these findings.

Differential Diagnosis

See Table 8-3, earlier. If retinal detachment is a presenting finding, other causes of infantile retinal detachment should be considered.

Diagnostic Evaluation

Typical fundus findings are noted on ophthalmoscopy. If FEVR is suspected, examination of the peripheral retina of asymptomatic family members may reveal findings consistent with the diagnosis.

Prognosis and Management

Patients who are affected at a young age usually have more severe pathology. Laser photocoagulation or cryotherapy to the peripheral avascular retina may prevent progression of fibrovascular complications. Scleral buckling and vitrectomy surgery have been attempted for more severe cases with retinal detachment. All family members of an affected individual should be examined, because progressive changes may occur throughout life.

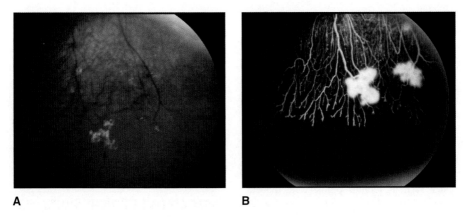

Figure 8-17 FEVR *A. Clinical photograph showing peripheral retinal capillary nonperfusion with some intraretinal lipid exudate* (arrow). ***B.** Corresponding fluorescein angiogram documenting peripheral nonperfusion and areas of neovascularization.*

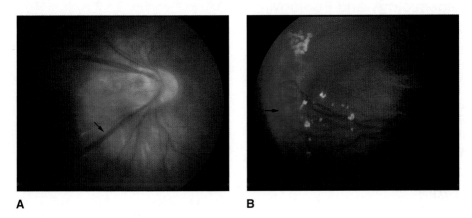

Figure 8-18 FEVR *A. Temporal dragging of the retina with vascular straightening* (arrow). *Compare with ROP, **Figure 8-8.** **B.** Temporal periphery with intraretinal lipid, peripheral retinal capillary nonperfusion, and peripheral neovascularization* (arrow).

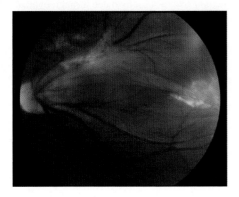

Figure 8-19 FEVR *Severe tractional retinal detachment with dragging.*

COATS' DISEASE

Definition

Coats' disease is a unilateral, idiopathic retinal vascular abnormality first described by George Coats in 1908. It is characterized by telangiectatic retinal vascular abnormalities in association with lipid exudation. Coats' disease should be differentiated from a *Coats' response,* or a large degree of lipid exudation, which can occur with abnormalities such as retinitis pigmentosa, diabetic retinopathy, retinal venous obstruction, retinal capillary hemangioma, and the late sequelae of retinopathy of prematurity.

Epidemiology and Etiology

Coats' disease is idiopathic. Most cases are diagnosed before age 20 with the peak incidence at the end of the first decade. It occurs predominately in males (85%) and is almost always uniocular. The severity of the disease varies widely from asymptomatic patches of telangiectatic vessels in the retinal periphery (Figure 8-20A,B) to total exudative retinal detachment (Figure 8-21).

History

Infants may present with strabismus, leukokoria, or a red, painful eye (from neovascular glaucoma). The severity and rate of progression are greatest in younger patients (less than 4 years of age). Older children and, rarely, adults may complain of reduced vision in one eye.

Pathophysiology

The retinal vessels become telangiectatic and develop multiple aneurysmal abnormalities. These can occur on the retinal arterial or venous sides, or both. Marked hard exudation is frequently present, extending from the retina into the subretinal space when it is massive.

Important Clinical Signs

Telangiectatic vessels, venous dilation, microaneurysms, and fusiform capillary dilation are the hallmark findings of Coats' disease (Figure 8-22). Progressive exudation from these retinal vascular abnormalities may lead to exudative retinal detachment.

Associated Clinical Signs

Posterior segment neovascularization is rare even though retinal capillary nonperfusion is often present. Retinal telangiectasis has been reported in association with many other ocular and systemic diseases. Retinitis pigmentosa with a "Coats'-like response" has been documented. Other entities associated with retinal telangiectasia are Alport's syndrome, tuberous sclerosis, Turner's syndrome, Senior-Loken syndrome, the ichthyosis hystrix variant of epidermal nevus syndrome, muscular dystrophy, and fascioscapulohumeral dystrophy.

Differential Diagnosis

The differential diagnosis of Coats' disease depends on the severity of the disease being considered (Table 8-5).

Diagnostic Evaluation

The diagnosis is usually made through ophthalmoscopy; however, fluorescein angiography may be helpful in detecting telangiectatic retinal vascular abnormalities. Characteristic "light-bulb" aneurysmal dilations of larger retinal vessels are particularly obvious on fluorescein angiography (Figure 8-23). Retinal capillary nonperfusion may also be seen with fluorescein angiography.

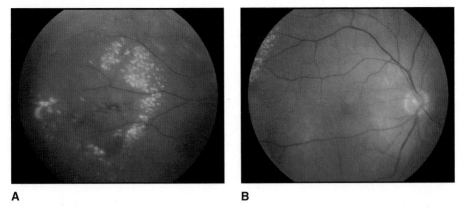

Figure 8-20   Coats' disease   *A. Peripheral fundus of an asymptomatic patient with micro-aneurysms, intraretinal hemorrhages, and lipid exudates.* **B.** *Posterior pole of the same patient with a normal macula.*

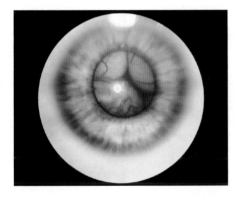

Figure 8-21   Coats' disease   *Total exudative retinal detachment.*

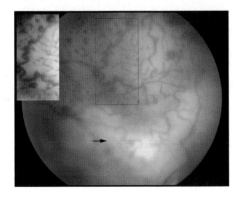

Figure 8-22   Coats' disease   *Peripheral fundus demonstrating venous dilation, microaneurysms, subretinal lipid exudation* (arrow), *and larger retinal vessels with "lightbulb" aneurysmal dilations* (inset).

TABLE 8-5   DIFFERENTIAL DIAGNOSIS OF COATS' DISEASE

Childhood Disease (Leukokoria or Exudative Retinal Detachment)

Retinoblastoma
Persistent hyperplastic primary vitreous/persistent fetal vasculature
Retinopathy of prematurity
Familial exudative vitreoretinopathy
Norrie's disease
Ocular toxocariasis
Von Hippel-Lindau disease
Peripheral exudative vitreoretinopathy
Incontinentia pigmenti (Bloch-Sulzberger syndrome)
Pars planitis
Retinitis pigmentosa with Coats'-like response
Vitreous hemorrhage

Parafoveal Telangiectasia with or without Lipid Exudation

Diabetic retinopathy
Radiation retinopathy
Juxtafoveal retinal telangiectasia
Branch retinal vein occlusion

Localized Telangiectasia with Arterial or Venous Aneurysms

Retinal cavernous hemangioma
Acquired retinal arterial macroaneurysm
Idiopathic retinal vasculitis, aneurysms, and neuroretinitis (IRVAN)

From Mandava N, Yannuzzi L. Miscellaneous retinal vascular conditions: Coats' disease. In Regillo CD, Brown GC, Flynn Jr HW (eds). Vitreoretinal Disease: The Essentials. New York, Thieme, 1999, p 196.

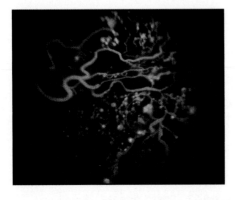

Figure 8-23   Coats' disease *Fluorescein angiogram of the same patient as in **Figure 8-22** clearly showing dilated retinal vessels with aneurysmal dilations.*

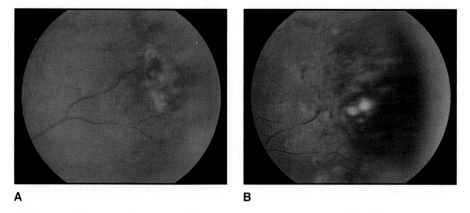

A   **B**

Figure 8-24   Coats' disease   *A. Peripheral fundus showing aneurysmal dilation and hemorrhage with some exudation from Coats' disease. **B.** Same area 4 months after cryotherapy showing involution of aneurysms and resolution of hemorrhage and exudates.*

Prognosis and Management

Management consists of observation; cryotherapy or laser photocoagulation may be applied to areas of retinal vascular abnormalities with progressive exudation (Figure 8-24A,B). Multiple treatment sessions are often necessary and close followup is warranted because recurrences have been reported up to 5 years after complete resolution. Vitrectomy and scleral buckling can be considered for retinal detachment.

CHORIORETINAL COLOBOMA

Definition

A chorioretinal coloboma is a developmental abnormality caused by failure of complete closure of the embryonic fissure.

Epidemiology and Etiology

Chorioretinal coloboma is a congenital developmental abnormality. There are rare cases of autosomal-recessive inheritance.

The retina and choroid are absent in areas affected. A thin intercalary membrane covers the sclera. This membrane consists of rudimentary retina with blood vessels. The coloboma is located inferiorly, because the embryonic fissure is located inferonasally in the developing eye.

History

Patients are usually asymptomatic unless the optic nerve or macula are involved or if there are secondary effects. Retinal breaks may occur in the intercalary membrane. Retinal detachment may then occur and cause symptoms.

Important Clinical Signs

A white area (sclera) is visible in the inferior fundus to a variable extent depending on the size of the defect (Figure 8-25). The margins of the coloboma are well defined. There is often a pigmented border marking the transition from the coloboma to the normal retina and choroid.

Associated Clinical Signs

The coloboma may extend back to the optic nerve (Figure 8-26) and forward to involve the ciliary body, zonule, and iris. The lens may be flattened at the pole corresponding to the coloboma owing to the missing zonule (Figure 8-27).

Differential Diagnosis

Chorioretinal scar (e.g., ocular toxoplasmosis)
Degenerative myopia

Diagnostic Evaluation

Ophthalmoscopy usually suffices to make the diagnosis of chorioretinal coloboma.

Prognosis and Management

No treatment is necessary unless retinal detachment occurs (Figure 8-28A,B). Vitrectomy surgery is necessary to manage the retinal detachment associated with chorioretinal coloboma. Internal drainage through the hole in the intercalary membrane is performed (if the hole can be found) and laser photocoagulation is placed around the margins of the coloboma.

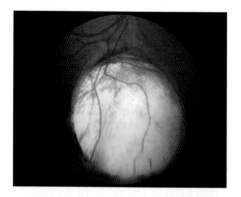

Figure 8-25 Chorioretinal coloboma
Chorioretinal defect in the inferior fundus.

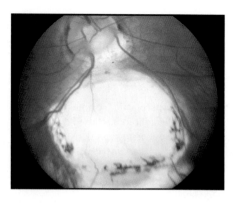

Figure 8-26 Chorioretinal coloboma
Colobomatous defect involving the inferior fundus and optic nerve.

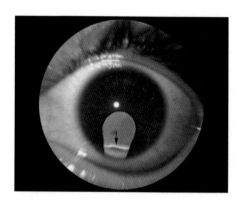

Figure 8-27 Chorioretinal coloboma
Extension of coloboma anteriorly. Note flattening of the inferior pole of the lens (arrow) *due to the missing portion of the zonule.*

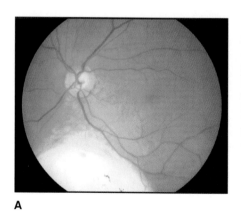

A

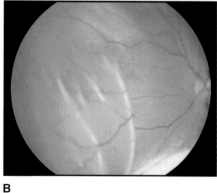

B

Figure 8-28 Chorioretinal coloboma *Posterior pole (A) and inferonasal area (B) of a patient with chorioretinal coloboma and associated rhegmatogenous retinal detachment.*

PERSISTENT HYPERPLASTIC PRIMARY VITREOUS/PERSISTENT FETAL VASCULATURE

Definition

Persistent hyperplastic primary vitreous (PHPV) was thought to be caused by failure of the primary vitreous to regress. Now the term *persistent fetal vasculature* (PFV) has been proposed to integrate the findings that occur when there is failure of regression of components of the fetal vessels.

Epidemiology and Etiology

Persistent hyperplastic primary vitreous/persistent fetal vasculature is a rare developmental abnormality. The condition is almost always unilateral and is more common in males than females. Anterior and posterior forms exist, and both may be present together.

History

In the anterior form infants present with leukokoria due to a white, vascularized fibrous membrane behind the lens. In the posterior form the eye may be microphthalmic but the anterior segment is otherwise normal. The infant may present with leukokoria due to a persistent stalk of tissue from the optic nerve to the retrolental region.

Important Clinical Signs

In the anterior form microphthalmia, a shallow anterior chamber and long ciliary processes visible through the pupil are seen in association with the white pupillary reflex (Figure 8-29). In the posterior form, the eye may be microphthalmic with a clear lens and no retrolental membrane. There is a stalk of tissue emanating from the optic disc to the retrolental area (Figure 8-30). Often, an associated retinal fold is located in an inferior quadrant.

Associated Clinical Signs

Cataract and narrow-angle glaucoma may occur in the anterior form of PFV if a dehiscence in the lens capsule occurs. Severe cases may progress to retinal detachment and phthisis bulbi.

Differential Diagnosis

The differential diagnosis of anterior PFV is that of leukokoria. The differential diagnosis of posterior PFV is ROP, ocular toxocariasis, and FEVR.

Diagnostic Evaluation

Clinical examination of the anterior segment is important in establishing the diagnosis of PFV. If the anterior segment is not affected, the diagnosis of posterior PFV can be established by ophthalmoscopy. Ultrasonography and computed tomographic (CT) scanning may help differentiate PFV from retinoblastoma, especially when the anterior segment is involved.

Prognosis and Management

Pars plana vitrectomy, lensectomy removal of the fibrovascular retrolental membrane, and anterior vitrectomy in anterior PFV help prevent narrow-angle glaucoma, but visual results are poor.

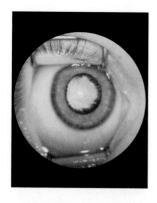

Figure 8-29   Persistent hyperplastic primary vitreous (PHPV)/persistent fetal vasculature (PFV)   *Anterior PHPV/PFV in a microphthalmic eye. Note the white reflex due to vascularized membrane behind the lens and ciliary processes dragged in toward the center.*

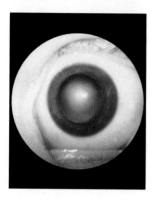

Figure 8-30   PHPV/PFV   *External view of posterior PHPV/PFV. Note termination of the stalk of tissue on the posterior surface of the lens. Ciliary processes are not dragged in toward the center.*

JUVENILE X-LINKED RETINOSCHISIS

Definition

Juvenile X-linked retinoschisis is a hereditary disorder characterized by diffuse retinal dysfunction with a stellate macula in all cases and splitting of the nerve fiber layer in 50% of cases.

Epidemiology and Etiology

Juvenile X-linked retinoschisis is a bilateral inherited disorder occurring in males. Linkage studies have localized the retinoschisis gene to the distal short arm of the X chromosome (Xp22.1-p22.3). The electroretinographic abnormalities implicate Müller cell dysfunction.

History

Patients may present with reduced vision from the macular changes. Earlier presentation occurs due to routine examination of family members with a family history of the disease. In patients with severe peripheral involvement, vitreous hemorrhage resulting from rupture of unsupported retinal vessels in the elevated nerve fiber layer may cause abrupt loss of vision.

Important Clinical Signs

Foveal schisis is present in all cases and appears as a stellate maculopathy on ophthalmoscopic examination (Figure 8-31A,B). The stellate appearance often gives way to ill-defined retinal pigment epithelial alterations in older patients.

Peripheral retinoschisis is present in 50% of patients (Figure 8-32). It is most common inferiorly and is at the level of the nerve fiber layer. Often, breaks occur in the elevated nerve fiber layer leaving unsupported retinal vessels that can rupture, causing vitreous hemorrhage (Figure 8-33). Breaks can occur in the inner layer causing rhegmatogenous retinal detachment (Figure 8-34).

Associated Clinical Signs

Less common findings include traction or exudative retinal detachment, extension of the retinoschisis into the macula, macular ectopia with nasal or temporal dragging, hypermetropia, cataract, and strabismus.

Differential Diagnosis

Retinopathy of prematurity
Goldmann-Favre disease
Retinitis pigmentosa
Familial exudative vitreoretinopathy

Diagnostic Evaluation

The stellate macula is often best seen with red-free illumination. Although it has the appearance of cystoid macular edema, there is no leakage of dye on fluorescein angiography. Electroretinography is useful because patients typically have selective loss of the b-wave. Examination of family members, some of whom may have the disease, may aid in diagnosis.

Prognosis and Management

There is no treatment for the macular aspects of the disease. Vitrectomy can be performed for nonclearing vitreous hemorrhage. Retinal detachment repair can be attempted with scleral buckling or vitrectomy techniques. Genetic counseling should be offered.

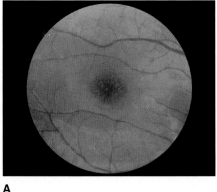

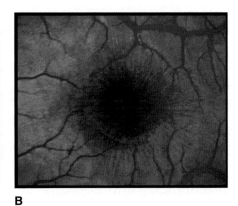

A

B

Figure 8-31   Juvenile X-linked retinoschisis   *A. Foveal schisis. **B.** High-power image of foveal schisis; note radiating retinal striae.*

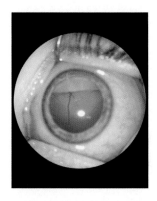

Figure 8-32   Juvenile X-linked retinoschisis   *Highly bullous peripheral retinoschisis.*

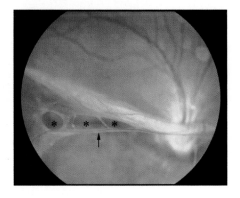

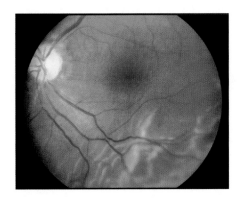

Figure 8-33   Juvenile X-linked retinoschisis   *Inferior retinoschisis with large breaks* (arrow) *and unsupported retinal vessels* (*).

Figure 8-34   Juvenile X-linked retinoschisis   *Rhegmatogenous retinal detachment in a patient with juvenile X-linked retinoschisis. Note the stellate appearance in the macula due to foveal schisis.*

LEBER'S CONGENITAL AMAUROSIS

Definition

Leber's congenital amaurosis is a group of diseases characterized by severe loss of vision from birth associated with nystagmus and severely impaired electroretinogram (ERG) responses for both rods and cones.

Epidemiology and Etiology

Leber's congenital amaurosis is a hereditary disease most commonly inherited as an autosomal-recessive trait. Several genetic defects have been identified.

History

Patients usually present because of nystagmus or strabismus; however, parents may be concerned earlier that the infant does not recognize faces.

Important Clinical Signs

The fundi are usually normal. Horizontal nystagmus is present.

Associated Clinical Signs

Many children are highly hyperopic. Older children may develop cataracts and keratoconus.

Differential Diagnosis

Albinism
Congenital stationary night blindness
Achromatopsia

Diagnostic Evaluation

Fundus examination is often not helpful because infants may have a normal-appearing fundus. Arteriolar attenuation, optic nerve pallor, and pigmentary degeneration may occur later in childhood (Figure 8-35). Electrophysiologic testing is necessary to establish a diagnosis. The ERG is typically minimal or extinguished.

Prognosis and Management

There is no treatment available.

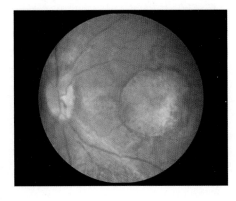

Figure 8-35   Leber's congenital amaurosis *Fundus of an older child demonstrating one of the late patterns of Leber's congenital amaurosis. Note pigmentary retinopathy and "macular coloboma," chorioretinal degeneration in the macula.*

Chapter 9

TRAUMATIC AND TOXIC RETINOPATHIES

J. Luigi Borrillo, MD

Carl D. Regillo, MD

COMMOTIO RETINAE

Definition

Commotio retinae is retinal whitening that occurs after blunt ocular trauma. This transient condition affects the outer retina. Often the damage incurred to the photoreceptors is reversible.

Epidemiology

Statistically the condition is most common in young males.

History

Patients have a history of blunt ocular trauma.

Clinical Signs

The condition is usually asymptomatic. Decreased vision may occur with macular involvement. The retina appears whitened, while the retinal vasculature remains unaffected. The retina regains its normal appearance within weeks (Figure 9-1A,B). Occasionally, changes to the retinal pigment epithelium (RPE), such as stippling or clumping, may be seen after the retinal whitening resolves.

Be mindful of other findings seen in trauma such as hyphema or microhyphema, choroidal rupture, retinal hemorrhage, retinal dialysis, avulsed vitreous base, and vitreous hemorrhage.

Differential Diagnosis

Other entities that may mimic commotio retinae include branch retinal artery occlusion, white-without-pressure, and shallow retinal detachment.

Diagnostic Evaluation

Diagnosis is based on clinical examination.

Prognosis and Management

Retinal whitening resolves without visual compromise. However, permanent visual acuity loss can sometimes occur if macular retinal pigment epithelial disruption is present.

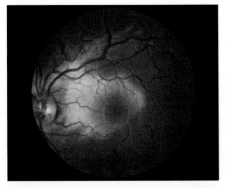

A

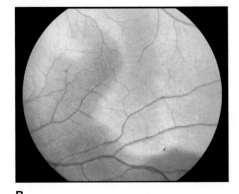

B

Figure 9-1   Commotio retinae
*A. Commotio retinae: Outer retinal whitening
in the posterior pole after blunt trauma.
B. Outer retinal whitening in the peripheral
retina. (B, Courtesy of Dr. Alexander
J. Brucker.)*

CHOROIDAL RUPTURE

Definition

In this injury, disruption of the choriocapillaris and Bruch's membrane occurs secondary to traumatic ocular compression. Ruptures located in the posterior pole are concentric to the optic disc. These breaks are often associated with subretinal and subretinal pigment epithelial hemorrhage.

Epidemiology and Etiology

Choroidal rupture occurs as a result of trauma, most commonly in young males.

History

Patients have a history of blunt ocular trauma.

Clinical Signs

The characteristic finding is subretinal hemorrhage, with whitish, crescent-shaped lesions around the optic disc (Figure 9-2A). In the acute setting, choroidal ruptures may be associated with other findings from blunt ocular trauma such as hyphema, iris sphincter ruptures, commotio retinae, vitreous hemorrhage, retinal tears, retinal dialysis, and orbital fractures. Later, choroidal neovascularization (CNV) may occur at the edge of the rupture site (Figure 9-2B).

Differential Diagnosis

Myopic lacquer cracks and angioid streaks may have a similar appearance. Other causes of subretinal hemorrhage include CNV, retinal arterial macroaneurysm, Valsalva retinopathy, and anemia.

Diagnostic Evaluation

Diagnosis is based on clinical examination.

Prognosis and Management

Visual prognosis depends on the location of the choroidal rupture with respect to the fovea and any associated subretinal or subretinal pigment epithelial hemorrhage. Secondary CNV can occur at anytime during the followup period and can cause visual acuity loss.

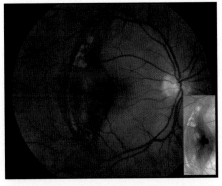

A

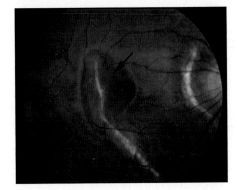

B

Figure 9-2 Choroidal rupture

A. Choroidal rupture: Crescent-shaped lesion in the macula with subretinal hemorrhage (inset). *B. Chronic choroidal rupture: Yellow crescent-shaped rupture site with pigmented choroidal neovascularization* (arrow) *and associated subretinal fluid in the fovea.*

AVULSED VITREOUS BASE

Definition

This entity describes separation of the vitreous base at the ora serrata that occurs secondary to trauma. Sometimes the avulsed vitreous base can be seen floating in the periphery.

Epidemiology and Etiology

The injury occurs as a result of trauma, usually in young males.

History

Patients have a history of blunt ocular trauma.

Clinical Signs

A semi-transparent, sometimes pigmented, curvilinear ribbon-like structure may or may not be completely separated from the retinal periphery (Figure 9-3). The presence of an avulsed vitreous base is pathognomonic for ocular trauma.

An avulsed vitreous base may be associated with hyphema, iris sphincter tears, commotio retinae, vitreous hemorrhage, retinal tears, retinal dialysis, or orbital fractures.

Differential Diagnosis

Avulsed vitreous base should be distinguished from retinal dialysis. Other entities that may mimic this condition include old vitreous hemorrhage.

Diagnostic Evaluation

Diagnosis is based on binocular indirect ophthalmoscopy with scleral depression.

Prognosis and Management

No treatment is necessary. Patients should be observed for the subsequent development of trauma-related ocular problems such as retinal breaks and angle-recession glaucoma.

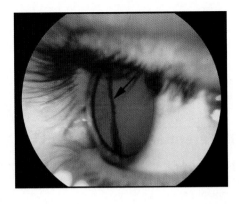

Figure 9-3 Avulsed vitreous base *Nasal avulsed vitreous base* (arrow) *is pathognomonic for prior trauma.*

SOLAR MACULOPATHY

Definition

Solar maculopathy is visual loss resulting from foveal photoreceptor and retinal pigment epithelial damage as a consequence of sun-gazing or direct observation of a solar eclipse.

Epidemiology

There is a trend for higher incidence in areas where a solar eclipse was directly observable. Solar maculopathy is more common among individuals involved in sun-worshiping religious groups. Loss of the ozone layer has been associated with solar retinopathy among sunbathers in the United States.

History

Patients have a history of sun gazing.

Clinical Signs

There is an abnormal foveal reflex. Often, a sharply demarcated yellow or reddish spot is visible in the fovea (Figure 9-4A–C). Retinal pigment epithelial changes (focal hyperpigmentation) may be evident in the foveal or parafoveal area at later stages.

Differential Diagnosis

Pseudomacular hole, photic maculopathy, and macular dystrophy or degeneration may have a similar appearance.

Diagnostic Evaluation

Diagnosis is based on clinical examination. Fluorescein angiography will reveal nonspecific retinal pigment epithelial window defects centered on the fovea.

Prognosis and Management

Good visual recovery occurs in most patients, but it may take weeks or months for vision to improve. No treatment is needed.

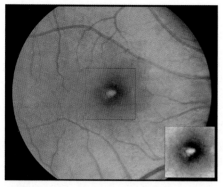

A

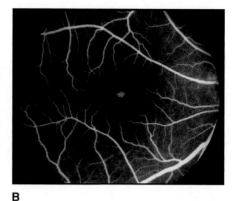

B

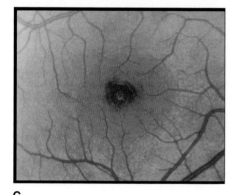

C

Figure 9-4   Solar retinopathy
*A. Color fundus photograph demonstrating
deep yellow foveal lesion* (inset). ***B.*** *Corresponding fluorescein angiogram photograph
demonstrating foveal window defect.* ***C.*** *Acute
solar retinopathy with yellow foveal lesion
and hemorrhage. Visual acuity is 20/30.
(****B,*** *Courtesy of Dr. Alexander
J. Brucker.)*

VALSALVA RETINOPATHY

Definition

In Valsalva retinopathy, unilateral or bilateral retinal or preretinal hemorrhage occurs as a result of an acute episode of increased intrathoracic pressure. Superficial capillaries rupture secondary to a sharp rise in ocular intravenous pressure.

Epidemiology

The condition can occur in persons of any age.

History

Patients usually have a history of recent strenuous physical exertion, coughing, vomiting, or straining (e.g., with constipation).

Clinical Signs

Single or multiple intraretinal hemorrhages (often underneath the internal limiting membrane) are noted in the posterior pole (Figure 9-5). There may be a decrease in visual acuity when the hemorrhage is localized in or over the foveal region.

Subconjunctival hemorrhage may be associated with this condition. Significant vitreous hemorrhage is rare.

Differential Diagnosis

Retinal macroaneurysm, diabetic retinopathy, venous occlusion, anemia, anticoagulant therapy, retinal tear, or posterior vitreous detachment with associated hemorrhage may mimic the findings of Valsalva retinopathy.

Diagnostic Evaluation

Diagnosis is based on clinical examination. B-scan ultrasonography is performed to evaluate for underlying retinal detachment or retinal tear in the setting of dense vitreous hemorrhage.

Prognosis and Management

The visual prognosis is good. Management consists of observation, only, in most cases. Hemorrhages will resolve spontaneously. Vitrectomy may be considered for nonclearing vitreous hemorrhage (but is rarely indicated).

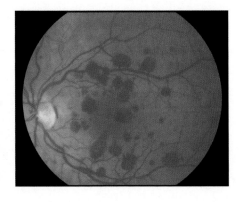

Figure 9-5 Valsalva retinopathy
Multiple superficial retinal hemorrhages in the macula.

SHAKEN BABY SYNDROME

Definition

This condition refers to intraocular hemorrhages in infants or young children secondary to child abuse. The findings are associated with decreased visual acuity and increased mortality.

Epidemiology

The condition is most common in infants and toddlers.

History

Recent, often multiple episodes of violent shaking of the infant precede findings, although it is often difficult to obtain a history of abuse from the caretaker. Caretakers may refuse diagnostic evaluation.

Clinical Signs

Subretinal, intraretinal, or preretinal hemorrhages are noted in one or (more commonly) both eyes (Figure 9-6A). The preretinal hemorrhages are typically globular as opposed to flat (Figure 9-6B). Other signs include poor visual or pupillary response. No single ocular finding is pathognomonic.

Ecchymosis, long bone and rib fractures, lethargy, or developmental delay are common associated findings. Often the child has physical findings that do not match the reported mechanism of the injuries.

Differential Diagnosis

Birth trauma—intraretinal hemorrhages may be seen in newborns, especially with the use of forceps in the delivery. These hemorrhages resolve over the course of weeks and are often not associated with neurologic sequelae.

Leukemia and intraocular infections may also mimic the ocular findings of shaken baby syndrome.

Diagnostic Evaluation

Clinical examination—evaluation for delayed neurologic development and systemic signs of child abuse

Head CT—to evaluate for intracranial hemorrhage

Bone scan—is more sensitive in detecting fractures and exposes the child to less radiation while providing a whole body skeletal survey. Bone scan findings may tailor subsequent x-ray studies.

X-ray studies—fractures at different stages of healing, leg fractures prior to bipedal ambulation (prior to 12 months of age), and posterior rib fractures are highly suspicious for child abuse.

Prognosis and Management

A pediatric consultation should be considered to evaluate for child abuse. The prognosis is largely dependent on associated brain injury. Poor pupillary response, poor visual acuity, and retinal hemorrhages have been associated with high infant mortality. Conversely, the presence of good visual acuity and normal pupillary reflexes are associated with a better prognosis.

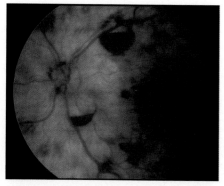

A

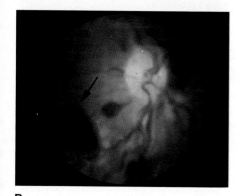

B

Figure 9-6   Shaken baby syndrome
*A. Multiple intraretinal and preretinal
hemorrhages in the posterior pole. **B.** Note
the globular nature* (arrows) *of the preretinal
hemorrhage in shaken baby syndrome.
(**A**, Courtesy of Dr. Richard Spaide.)*

TERSON'S SYNDROME

Definition

Terson's syndrome encompasses any intraocular (usually preretinal or vitreous) hemorrhage associated with either trauma-induced or spontaneous acute intracranial bleeding.

Epidemiology and Etiology

The syndrome may affect individuals of any age. The sudden increase in intracranial pressure directly or indirectly ruptures the peripapillary capillaries.

History

The presentation may include severe headache or known acute neurologic event.

Clinical Signs

Patients may have varying degrees of decreased visual acuity and multiple, usually bilateral, retinal hemorrhages (Figure 9-7A,B). Vitreous hemorrhage can also occur and may be dense. Other ocular signs associated with Terson's syndrome include cranial nerve palsies, late-appearing epiretinal membrane, or tractional retinal detachment.

The intracranial hemorrhages are usually located in the subarachnoid space. Spontaneous hemorrhages are a result of vascular abnormalities such as aneurysms, arteriovenous malformations, or fistulas.

Differential Diagnosis

Posterior vitreous detachment with vitreous hemorrhage, retinal vein occlusion, retinal tear, proliferative diabetic retinopathy, Valsalva retinopathy, or retinal arterial macroaneurysm may mimic Terson's syndrome.

Diagnostic Evaluation

Neuroimaging is performed, using computed tomography [CT] or magnetic resonance imaging [MRI]. B-scan ultrasonography is used to evaluate for retinal detachment or retinal tear in cases where vitreous hemorrhage precludes a view of the posterior segment.

Prognosis and Management

The visual prognosis is often good. There can be a high mortality rate depending on the location and severity of the intracranial hemorrhage. Neurosurgical consultation is recommended. In cases of bilateral vitreous hemorrhage or dense nonclearing vitreous hemorrhage, vitrectomy may be considered.

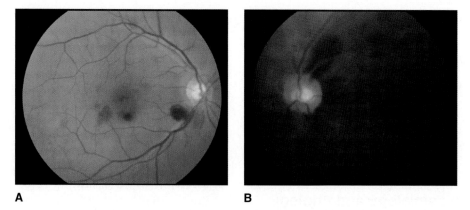

Figure 9-7 Terson's syndrome *A. Multiple retinal and preretinal hemorrhages in the posterior pole of a patient who has suffered an acute subarachnoid hemorrhage. **B.** More severe retinal hemorrhaging and vitreous hemorrhage in Terson's syndrome.*

PURTSCHER'S RETINOPATHY

Definition

Purtscher's retinopathy describes decreased vision associated with intraretinal hemorrhages and patches of retinal whitening secondary to severe crushing injuries to the torso or head. The fundus findings are concentrated in the peripapillary area and may be unilateral or bilateral.

Epidemiology and Etiology

Persons of any age may be affected. Endothelial damage leads to intravascular coagulopathy and granulocytic aggregation with microemboli formation.

History

There is a history of compressive trauma.

Clinical Signs

Acutely, severe vision loss is noted in one or both eyes. Cotton-wool spots centered on the optic disc, hemorrhages, exudates, and retinal edema are often seen. Fundus findings resolve over several weeks (Figure 9-8A). Optic atrophy may be a late finding.

Differential Diagnosis

This condition should be distinguished from Purtscher's-like retinopathy, which has a similar fundus presentation associated with microemboli of various compositions from a wide spectrum of systemic conditions such as pancreatitis, amniotic fluid embolism, collagen vascular disease, thrombotic thrombocytopenic purpura, and long bone fractures (Figure 9-8B).

Central retinal artery and vein occlusion may also mimic the findings of Purtscher's retinopathy.

Diagnostic Evaluation

CT imaging of chest and long bones is performed, when indicated. Fluorescein angiography typically reveals areas of retinal ischemia.

Prognosis and Management

Permanent visual loss may occur in half of affected patients. No treatment is available.

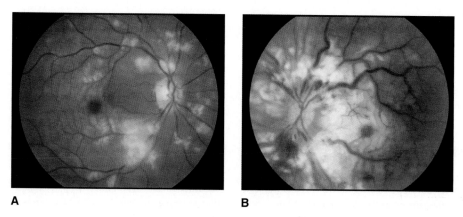

A   B

Figure 9-8   Purtscher's retinopathy   *A. Purtscher's retinopathy: Multiple peripapillary cotton-wool spots centered around the optic disc in a patient with massive chest trauma. B. Purtscher's-like retinopathy: Multiple cotton-wool spots, hemorrhage, and macular infarction in a woman with acute thrombotic thrombocytopenic purpura. (**B,** reproduced with permission from Power MH, Regillo CD, Custis PH. Thrombotic thrombocytopenic purpura associated with Purtscher retinopathy. Arch Ophthalmol 1997; 115:128–129.)*

TRAUMATIC MACULAR HOLE

Definition

This entity describes a full-thickness macular hole occurring after blunt ocular trauma.

Epidemiology and Etiology

Persons of any age may be affected. The foveal defect develops as a result of vitreous traction or contusion necrosis of the retina and may be a direct consequence of globe deformation.

History

There is a history of recent blunt trauma or whiplash injury.

Clinical Signs

A full-thickness macular hole with irregular border is seen on clinical examination. Macular pigmentary changes are often observed (Figure 9-9A,B), as well as a positive Watzke-Allen sign.

Other associated signs may include submacular hemorrhage, choroidal rupture, commotio retinae, or vitreous hemorrhage. The presence of a posterior vitreous detachment is unlikely.

Differential Diagnosis

Solar retinopathy
Nontraumatic macular hole
Pseudohole secondary to epiretinal membrane

Diagnostic Evaluation

Careful contact lens biomicroscopy is indicated. Fluorescein angiography may reveal a hyperfluorescent spot at the fovea corresponding to a retinal pigment epithelial defect. Optical coherence tomography will reveal full-thickness neurosensory retinal loss in the fovea.

Prognosis and Management

The visual prognosis is variable. Spontaneous closure of traumatic macular holes in young patients has been reported in the literature but is rare. A recent series suggests that macular hole surgery may be beneficial, with reported visual acuity of 20/50 or better in 64% of patients.

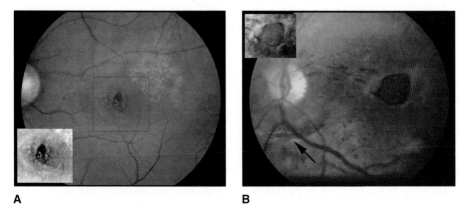

Figure 9-9 Traumatic macular hole *A. Small, irregular full-thickness macular hole* (inset) *and associated macular retinal pigment epithelial clumping.* ***B.*** *Larger, irregular traumatic macular hole* (inset) *with marked retinal pigment epithelial alterations and a choroidal rupture* (arrow) *inferior to the optic disc.*

CHORIORETINITIS SCLOPETARIA

Definition

Chorioretinitis sclopetaria is full-thickness disruption of the choroid and retina secondary to the concussive forces of a nonpenetrating high-velocity projectile.

Epidemiology and Etiology

The injury is most common in young males. Traveling at high speeds, the projectile creates shock waves that can rupture choroid and retina but leave sclera intact. The defects are subsequently replaced by fibrous tissue.

History

Patients have a history of a high-velocity projectile, such as a BB pellet, to the orbit.

Clinical Signs

The visual acuity is variable. Acutely, there may be preretinal, intraretinal, or subretinal hemorrhage as well as vitreous hemorrhage (Figure 9-10A). Subsequently, lesions have a "claw-like" branching pattern (Figure 9-10B). Bare sclera may be visible through the full-thickness defects of the choroid and overlying retina. Sclopetaria is usually located in the peripheral fundus, corresponding to the path of the projectile. Often these areas are covered by hemorrhage.

Fibrous proliferation at the rupture sites eventually ensues and becomes visible as any associated hemorrhage clears. Intraorbital foreign body is often present.

Differential Diagnosis

A ruptured globe should be ruled out. Choroidal ruptures may demonstrate a similar appearance as sclopetaria, but they are usually located in the posterior pole.

Diagnostic Evaluation

Computed tomographic imaging is important to evaluate the integrity of the globe, detect any associated orbital or central nervous system injuries, and identify any orbital foreign bodies.

Prognosis and Management

Visual prognosis is dependent on the location of sclopetaria. Lesions involving the macular region have poorer visual acuity.

Initial management is nonsurgical. The subsequent cicatricial process often fuses tissues, making retinal detachments unlikely. Surgery is indicated in the subsequent development of retinal detachment or for the removal of nonclearing vitreous hemorrhage.

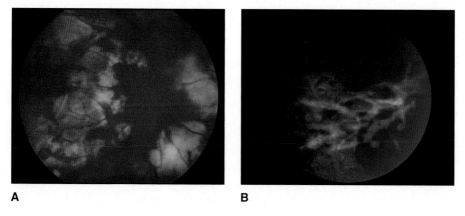

Figure 9-10   Chorioretinitis sclopetaria   *A. Retinal whitening and preretinal hemorrhage in the posterior pole of a patient sustaining an orbital foreign body injury. **B.** Claw-like chorioretinal scarring after a high-velocity bullet passed through the orbit adjacent to the eye.*

INTRAOCULAR FOREIGN BODY

Definition

Intraocular foreign body (IOFB) refers to the presence of a foreign body in the eye from a penetrating injury.

Epidemiology and Etiology

Young males are most commonly affected. The foreign body may serve as a nidus for endophthalmitis or severe inflammatory reaction. An IOFB may also cause delayed effects secondary to proliferative vitreoretinopathy or toxicity.

History

Most often there is a history of penetrating ocular injury. A foreign body sensation associated with hammering, grinding, or other mechanism of injury may also be elicited. Injury in a rural setting increases the risk of secondary endophthalmitis.

Clinical Signs

Visual acuity is variable. An obvious or subtle point of entry of the IOFB may be seen (Figure 9-11A). Other signs associated with IOFBs include sectorial microcystic corneal edema, irregular pupil, transillumination iris defect, low intraocular pressure, intraocular inflammation, or vitreous hemorrhages. Later findings include endophthalmitis, heterochromia, cataract, or corneal deposits.

Substances such as vegetable, iron, copper, and steel may lead to intense inflammation or infection. Nickel, aluminum, and mercury tend to produce mild inflammation. Glass, carbon, porcelain, silver, and platinum are inert.

Differential Diagnosis

Endophthalmitis and uveitis may mimic the findings of IOFB.

Diagnostic Evaluation

Orbital CT is the imaging modality of choice in detecting nonorganic IOFBs. Small organic foreign bodies such as wood or vegetable matter may escape detection. B-scan ultrasonography may detect IOFBs, retinal tears, or retinal detachments when the posterior pole cannot be visualized (Figure 9-11B). Serial electroretinograms should be considered for retained metallic foreign bodies to evaluate for toxic metallosis.

Prognosis and Management

Prognosis is largely dependent on the location and nature of the IOFB. Repair of the ruptured globe should be the first priority. Prompt removal of the IOFB via pars plana vitrectomy before 24 hours has been found to decrease the incidence of endophthalmitis. Table 9-1 summarizes several considerations in the management of IOFBs.

Prompt surgical removal is recommended for vegetable, copper, iron, steel, or inert substances with toxic chemical coatings. Surgical extraction of certain metallic IOFBs may be facilitated by a magnet.

Systemic and intravitreal antibiotics should be administered when there is a high index of suspicion for endophthalmitis.

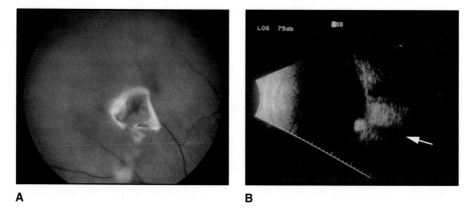

Figure 9-11   Intraocular foreign body   *A. Metallic foreign body in the retinal periphery.*
***B.** B-scan ultrasonography demonstrating acoustic shadowing* (arrow) *behind the intraocular foreign body.*

TABLE 9-1   **CONSIDERATIONS IN MANAGEMENT OF INTRAOCULAR
                 FOREIGN BODIES**

Always consider an intraocular foreign body masquerade syndrome in the setting of unilateral
   unexplained uveitis.

A CT scan with 1-mm sections through the globe and orbit is the best single imaging scan. MRI
   may be superior for imaging wood and organic material.

Copper, iron, and steel produce the most intense intraocular inflammatory response.

Surgical removal of intraocular foreign bodies is considered emergent and should be performed as
   soon as possible. Endophthalmitis associated with IOFBs is estimated up to 20%.

DISLOCATED LENS

Definition

This term describes the total displacement of the native lens into the anterior chamber or the vitreous cavity as a result of lens zonular disruption.

Epidemiology

The condition is most common in young males in the setting of trauma. Individuals with a familial or metabolic predisposition to zonular weakness are also prone to lens dislocation.

History

There is usually a history of blunt ocular trauma. Often, the patient notes a dramatic decrease in visual acuity because of lens malposition.

Clinical Signs

There is decreased vision, and the natural lens is seen in the anterior chamber or posterior pole (Figure 9-12). Other signs associated with lens dislocation may include iridodonesis, irregular anterior chamber depth, eyelid ecchymosis, vitreous hemorrhage, or orbital fractures.

The patient may have a physical habitus compatible with predisposing conditions such as Marfan's syndrome or Weill-Marchesani syndrome, among others.

Differential Diagnosis

Conditions other than severe blunt trauma that predispose patients to lens dislocation include:

Marfan's syndrome—patients are often tall and may have arachnodactyly. Cardiac evaluation is important in evaluation for aortic aneurysm or insufficiency.

Weill-Marchesani syndrome—affected individuals have short stature, seizures, microspherophakia, brachydactyly, and may have decreased hearing.

Homocystinuria—patients may have marfanoid features, thrombosis (especially with general anesthesia), and below-average IQ.

Other—syphilis, sulfite oxidase deficiency, high myopia, Ehlers-Danlos syndrome, and aniridia are other possible etiologies of lens dislocation.

Diagnostic Evaluation

B-scan ultrasonography is used in the setting of vitreous hemorrhage to evaluate for lens position and retinal detachment. Medical consultation is appropriate if Marfan's syndrome, homocystinuria, syphilis, or another predisposing condition is suspected.

Prognosis and Management

Conservative management such as observation and contact lens wear may be considered. Management of dislocation of the natural lens into the anterior chamber causing glaucoma may include a trial of pupillary dilation and supine positioning in an attempt to dislocate the lens into the vitreous cavity. A lens that cannot be repositioned into the vitreous cavity or that has a disrupted lens capsule may require vitrectomy and lensectomy.

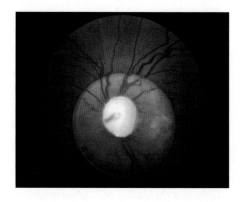

Figure 9-12   Dislocated lens   *Intact native lens in the vitreous over a glaucomatous optic disc. (Courtesy of the Wills Eye Hospital collection, Philadelphia, Pennsylvania.)*

TALC RETINOPATHY

Definition

Talc retinopathy describes the presence of an intraretinal, yellow, refractile substance in patients who abuse intravenous drugs, especially those using products made from crushed tablets or powder.

Epidemiology and Etiology

The condition can occur in persons of any age. The talc component of the injected medication migrates through microvascular venular to arteriolar shunts in the lung and into the retinal arterioles.

History

Patients have a history of chronic intravenous drug abuse. A history of intravenous injection of crushed methylphenidate (Ritalin) tablets may be elicited.

Clinical Signs

Irregular refractile elements are seen throughout the retina (intravascular space), especially within the macula (Figure 9-13A,B). Other intraocular signs that may be seen include neovascularization of the retinal periphery (or optic nerve), macular pucker or fibrosis, or vitreous hemorrhage. Inspection of the skin may reveal evidence of intravenous drug abuse.

Differential Diagnosis

The differential diagnosis for talc retinopathy includes other causes of crystalline retinopathy such as:

> *Canthaxanthine toxicity*—patients may volunteer a history of using oral tanning agents. The total cumulative dosage usually exceeds 19 g.
>
> *Tamoxifen (Nolvadex) use*—often there is a history of breast cancer and use of the antiestrogen agent for a cumulative dosage of at least 7.7 g.
>
> *Retinal emboli* associated with carotid obstructive disease or cardiac valve disease. Carotid ultrasonography or cardiac echography may reveal the embolic source.

See also Table 9-2.

Diagnostic Evaluation

Fluorescein angiography may reveal areas of nonperfusion in the retinal periphery.

Prognosis and Management

The visual prognosis is variable. In the setting of chronic intravenous drug abuse, visual acuity may be decreased as a result of macular retinal capillary nonperfusion or vitreous hemorrhage. Decreased visual acuity may also occur secondary to macular fibrosis associated with intravenous methylphenidate abuse. Peripheral laser treatment can cause regression of retinal neovascularization.

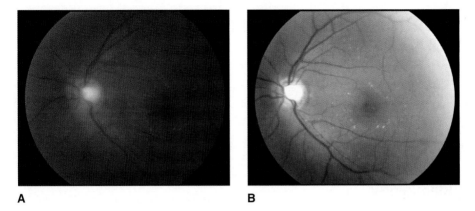

A   B

Figure 9-13   Talc retinopathy   *A. Color fundus photograph demonstrating yellow refractile particles within the retina.* **B.** *Red-free fundus photograph highlighting intraretinal macular refractile deposits.*

TABLE 9-2   **DIFFERENTIAL DIAGNOSIS: RETINAL CRYSTALS**

Intraretinal Crystals	Subretinal Crystals (often associated with RPE alterations)
Talc particles (intravenous drug abuse)	Calcific drusen (AMD)
Cholesterol (Hollenhorst plaque) or other emboli	Bietti's corneal and macular crystalline dystrophy
Canthaxanthine ingestion (oral tanning agent)	
Tamoxifen	
Methoxyflurane anesthesia	
Cystinosis	
Parafoveal telangectasia (Singerman's dots)	
Intraretinal lipid (hard exudates)	

AMD = age-related macular degeneration; RPE = retinal pigment epithelium.

CHLOROQUINE OR HYDROXYCHLOROQUINE RETINOPATHY

Definition

This entity describes degeneration of the RPE and neurosensory retinal damage resulting from chronic daily ingestion of chloroquine (Aralen) or hydroxychloroquine (Plaquenil).

Epidemiology

The condition occurs in individuals receiving chloroquine for antimalarial treatment and in patients with rheumatoid arthritis or lupus erythematosus who take hydroxychloroquine. Hydroxychloroquine is less likely than chloroquine to cause retinopathy.

History

There is a history of daily dosages exceeding 250 mg of chloroquine or 400 mg of hydroxychloroquine.

Clinical Signs

Visual acuity is variable. An abnormal foveal reflex and subtle parafoveal retinal pigment epithelial stippling precedes the development of a ring of retinal pigment epithelial atrophy surrounding the foveal region, known as the classic "bull's-eye" maculopathy (Figure 9-14A,B). Retinal pigment epithelial disturbance underneath the fovea is associated with decreased visual acuity. A paracentral scotoma is the earliest sign of chloroquine or hydroxychloroquine toxicity and may precede the development of fundus findings.

Other signs of chloroquine or hydroxychloroquine retinopathy include retinal vessel attenuation and corneal verticillata. Patients may display systemic findings of rheumatoid arthritis or lupus erythematosus.

Differential Diagnosis

Other conditions that may display a bull's-eye maculopathy include age-related macular degeneration (AMD), Stargardt's disease, cone dystrophy, and other conditions. See also Table 9-3.

Diagnostic Evaluation

Amsler grid evaluation may allow the patient to detect early scotoma formation. Humphrey visual field testing using red light may be the most sensitive means of detecting a paracentral scotoma. Color vision testing may reveal dyschromatopsia. Fluorescein angiography will show retinal pigment epithelial window defects in macular region. Electroretinography and electrooculography may be abnormal late findings.

Prognosis and Management

Prompt discontinuation of medication on detection of toxicity usually prevents further damage to the RPE and retina. Patients with mild retinal pigment epithelial changes may revert to normal and retain good visual acuity. However, in advanced cases, the condition may worsen despite cessation of the medication, and visual loss may ensue.

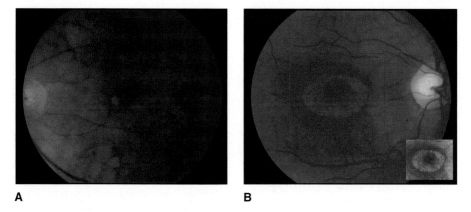

A   **B**

Figure 9-14   Chloroquine retinopathy   *A. Subtle parafoveal retinal pigment epithelial alterations* (arrow) *in a patient with a history of long-term chloroquine use.* ***B.*** *Bull's-eye maculopathy* (inset) *associated with chloroquine retinopathy. (****A****, Courtesy of Dr. Alexander J. Brucker;* ***B****, courtesy of the Wills Eye Hospital collection, Philadelphia, Pennsylvania.)*

TABLE 9-3   DIFFERENTIAL DIAGNOSIS: BULL'S-EYE MACULA

Cone dystrophy
Chloroquine or hydroxychloroquine toxicity
Benign concentric annular dystrophy
Spielmeyer-Vogt-Batten disease
Stargardt's maculopathy
Age-related macular degeneration
Fenestrated sheen macular dystrophy

THIORIDAZINE RETINOPATHY

Definition

Thioridazine retinopathy describes visual disturbance and pigmentary retinopathy that results from chronic high-dose thioridazine use. Daily doses are more predictive of retinal toxicity than total cumulative dose.

Epidemiology and Etiology

Individuals with psychiatric disorders requiring thioridazine. The exact mechanism of retinal damage is unclear although the medication is felt to accumulate in retinal pigment epithelial cells.

History

The use of thioridazine (Mellaril) in excess of 800 mg per day has been associated with retinopathy.

Clinical Signs

Acute toxicity is manifested by the sudden onset of visual disturbance, nyctalopia, or dyschromatopsia (red or brown coloration of vision). Retinal pigment epithelial changes can progress despite drug cessation. Early changes include granular retinal pigment epithelial stippling posterior to the equator. Nummular retinal pigment epithelial loss may be seen in intermediate stages (Figure 9-15A–C). Late features of thioridazine toxicity include optic atrophy, retinal vessel attenuation, diffuse RPE, and choriocapillaris atrophy.

Differential Diagnosis

Gyrate atrophy, retinitis pigmentosa, cancer-associated retinopathy, choroideremia, syphilis, viral chorioretinitis, and trauma may demonstrate findings similar to thioridazine toxicity.

Diagnostic Evaluation

Humphrey visual field testing may reveal paracentral scotomas or constriction. Fluorescein angiography may reveal a spectrum of retinal pigment epithelial window defects and disruption of the choriocapillaris. The electroretinogram may be normal in early stages, but demonstrate attenuation in later stages.

Prognosis and Management

Cessation of the drug early in the course of the toxicity may lead to reversal of visual disturbance. However, prolonged use of the medication may lead to progressive visual loss despite drug cessation.

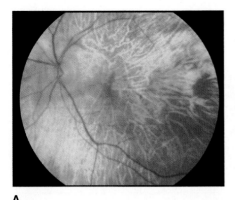

A

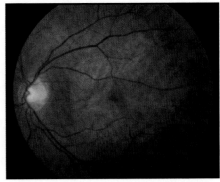

B

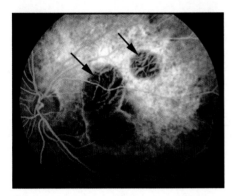

C

Figure 9-15 Thioridazine retinopathy
*A. Widespread retinal pigment epithelial and choriocapillaris atrophy. **B.** Less widespread retinal pigment epithelial and choriocapillaris atrophy may be mistaken for geographic atrophy due to age-related macular degeneration. Visual acuity is 20/200. **C.** Fluorescein angiogram showing retinal pigment epithelial atrophy as well as nummular areas of choroidal vascular loss* (arrows).

Chapter 10

PERIPHERAL RETINAL DISEASE

James F. Vander, MD

RETINAL BREAK OR TEAR

Definition

Retinal break or tear describes a full-thickness defect in the retina, generally in the retinal periphery, although the break may occur anywhere. Breaks occurring as the result of vitreous traction are known as retinal tears.

Epidemiology and Etiology

Retinal breaks are common. They are more frequent in myopia, pseudophakia, and after trauma. Many cases are bilateral and multiple. Retinal tears are caused by vitreous traction, most commonly found with degenerative vitreous liquefaction and posterior vitreous detachment (Figures 10-1 and 10-2). Other retinal breaks (see later discussion) result from developmental or degenerative abnormalities or trauma.

History

Retinal tears are often associated with floaters and flashing lights (photopsia). Many breaks are asymptomatic. If associated with retinal detachment, then progressive visual field loss occurs.

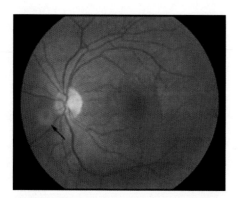

Figure 10-1 Posterior vitreous detachment (PVD) *Annulus of condensed vitreous (Weiss ring)* (arrow) *floating in front of the optic disc after PVD.*

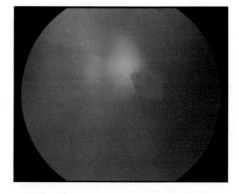

Figure 10-2 PVD *PVD (same patient as* **Figure 10-1***) focused on Weiss ring.*

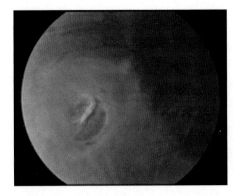

Figure 10-3   Retinal tear *Horseshoe tear with a few flecks of hemorrhage and a small amount of subretinal fluid surrounding it.*

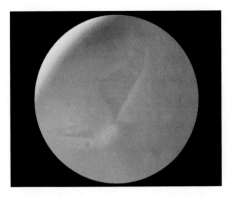

Figure 10-4   Retinal tear *Large horseshoe tear with a bridging retinal vessel.*

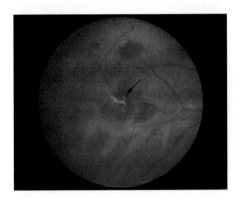

Figure 10-5   Retinal tear *Horseshoe tear with associated retinal hemorrhages* (arrow). *Vitreous elevates the flap tear.*

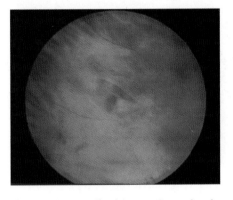

Figure 10-6   Retinal tear *Operculated retinal tear.*

Important Clinical Signs

Types of Retinal Breaks

Horseshoe (flap) tears—the horseshoe is open anteriorly. Vitreoretinal traction often persists (Figures 10-3 through 10-5).

Operculated tears—a fragment of retina is torn completely free of the retina and floats above it. The vitreous traction is relieved (Figure 10-6).

Atrophic retinal break—usually round, often small, holes; not associated with traction (Figure 10-7).

Retinal dialysis—disinsertion of the retina from the pars plana at the ora serrata; most often inferotemporal; superonasal is virtually pathognomonic for trauma (Figure 10-8).

Giant tear—a tear greater than 90 degrees, spontaneous or posttraumatic (Figure 10-9).

Stretch/necrotic tears—traumatic tears of variable size, often irregular in orientation with jagged edges; hemorrhage or other signs of trauma (Figures 10-10 through 10-12).

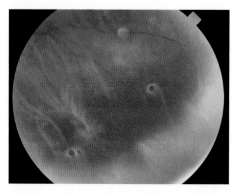

Figure 10-7 Peripheral cystoid degeneration *Peripheral cystoid degeneration with associated atrophic retinal holes.*

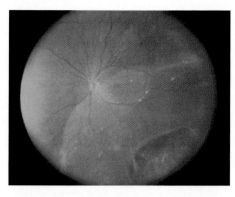

Figure 10-8 Retinal dialysis *Wide-angle view of inferotemporal dialysis with associated retinal detachment.*

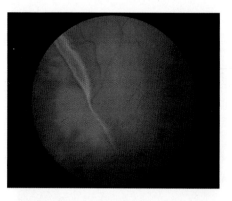

Figure 10-9 Giant retinal tear *Rolled edge of a giant retinal tear.*

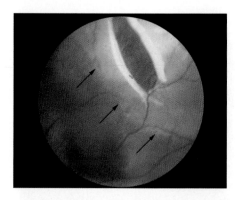

Figure 10-10 Posttraumatic retinal tear *Stretch tear after blunt trauma* (arrows *to retinal detachment*).

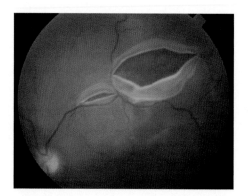

Figure 10-11 Posttraumatic retinal tear *Two stretch tears after blunt trauma.*

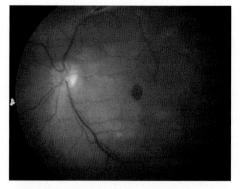

Figure 10-12 Posttraumatic macular hole *Traumatic macular hole.*

Associated Clinical Signs

Look for predisposing conditions (see earlier discussion)

Pigment cells in the vitreous ("tobacco dust")

Posterior vitreous detachment

Vitreous hemorrhage (tears are found in 70% of patients with hemorrhagic proliferative vitreoretinopathy)

Subretinal fluid accumulating around the tear

Pigment around the base of the retinal break (indicates chronicity)

Differential Diagnosis

Vitreoretinal tuft

Meridional fold or complex

Outer wall hole in retinoschisis

Cobblestone degeneration

Lattice degeneration

Diagnostic Evaluation

Indirect ophthalmoscopy with scleral depression is critical. Contact lens examination of the periphery may help confirm the presence and nature of the break.

Prognosis and Management

The risk of developing retinal detachment (and, therefore, indication for prophylactic treatment) depends on the type of break present. Symptomatic tears with persistent traction (horseshoe tears, giant tears) have a high risk of subsequent retinal detachment and are treated when recognized. Asymptomatic flap tears have a lower risk but are often prophylactically treated. Symptomatic operculated tears also have a much lower risk of subsequent retinal detachment. Treatment is more controversial. Dialysis and other posttraumatic tears are generally treated when recognized. Treatment for atrophic breaks, asymptomatic operculated tears, and breaks with pigment around them almost never require prophylactic treatment. Exceptions might include patients with a history of retinal detachment of the fellow eye, anticipated cataract surgery, or a strong family history of retinal tears or retinal detachment.

Treatment options include cryotherapy or laser photocoagulation (Figures 10-13 through 10-16). Development of the indirect ophthalmoscopic laser delivery system has facilitated the use of laser treatment and reduced the need for cryotherapy, which generally produces more pain during treatment. Patients with cloudy media or significant subretinal fluid may be better treated with cryotherapy.

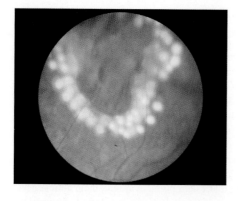

Figure 10-13 Retinal tear, posttreatment *Horseshoe retinal tear immediately after laser photocoagulation.*

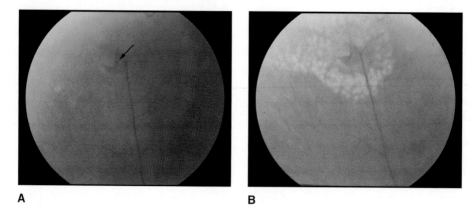

A

B

Figure 10-14 Retinal tear, pretreatment and posttreatment *A. Small horseshoe tear* (arrow). *B. Immediately after laser photocoagulation.*

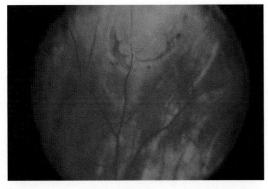

A

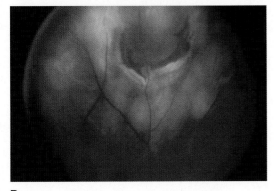

Figure 10-15   Retinal tear, pretreatment and posttreatment
A. Horseshoe tear with bridging vessel.
B. Immediately after laser photocoagulation.

B

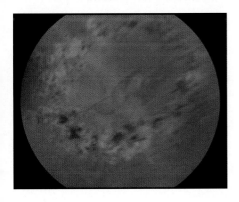

Figure 10-16   Retinal tear, posttreatment *Several weeks after laser photocoagulation for retinal tear. Laser marks have become pigmented.*

RHEGMATOGENOUS RETINAL DETACHMENT

Definition

Rhegmatogenous retinal detachment (RD) is a separation of the retina from the underlying retinal pigment epithelium (RPE) by fluid that gains access to the subretinal space via one or more full-thickness retinal breaks.

Epidemiology and Etiology

Epidemiology is the same as that for retinal breaks since, by definition, a retinal break is present and the cause of the RD. Retinal breaks develop into rhegmatogenous RD by a combination of vitreoretinal traction and fluid currents that cause vitreous fluid to move through the retinal break(s) and overcome the normal attractive forces between the photoreceptors and the RPE.

History

There is a progressive loss of the visual field (often described as a curtain or shadow blocking the vision), frequently accompanied or preceded by floaters and flashing lights. Patients with peripheral RDs may be asymptomatic or simply have flashes and floaters.

Important Clinical Signs

In addition to identifying the retinal break(s), the retina is seen to be elevated by subretinal fluid (Figures 10-17 through 10-19). The retina loses its transparency to a variable degree, often becoming translucent with a corrugated appearance. There is undulation with eye movement. Chronic rhegmatogenous RD may appear transparent and not undulate. Identifying the retinal break (often small and difficult to find) is the key. Pseudophakic retinal detachments are often caused by small, pinpoint retinal holes at the vitreous base and may be difficult to detect.

Associated Clinical Signs

Pigment—granules in the vitreous are almost always seen. Hyperpigmentation or loss of pigment at the RPE is common, especially in chronic RD. Linear pigment ("demarcation line") suggests chronicity and may be multiple (Figures 10-20 and 10-21).

Hypotony—relative to the fellow eye. This is not invariably present. In chronic rhegmatogenous RD, pressure may be normal or even high.

Other features of chronic RD—retinal neovascularization, cataract, anterior uveitis, rubeosis iridis, and retinal cysts (Figures 10-22 and 10-23).

Differential Diagnosis

Retinoschisis
Exudative RD
Tractional RD
Choroidal detachment

Diagnostic Evaluation

Indirect ophthalmoscopy with scleral depression is the key. Contact lens examination may help find small peripheral retinal breaks. Slit-lamp examination of the anterior vitreous confirms vitreous pigment. B-scan ultrasonography confirms retinal elevation in cases with media opacities. Examine the fellow eye to look for retinoschisis.

Prognosis and Management

Prognosis Chronic, asymptomatic RD may remain stationary and not require treatment. Spontaneous regression of RD can occur but is rare (Figure 10-24). Most RDs and virtually all symptomatic detachments will progress, causing severe permanent visual loss if untreated.

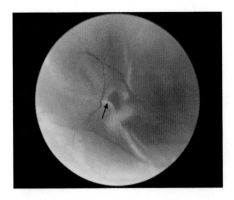

Figure 10-17   Rhegmatogenous retinal detachment (RD)   *Rhegmatogenous RD with a small horseshoe tear* (arrow).

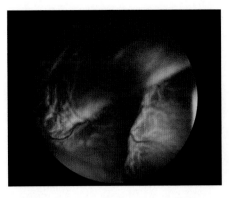

Figure 10-18   Rhegmatogenous RD   *RD with bullous elevation and corrugated appearance of the detached retina.*

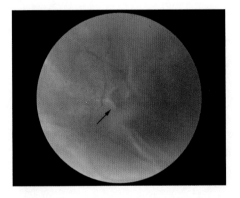

Figure 10-19   Rhegmatogenous RD   *RD with a small horseshoe tear* (arrow).

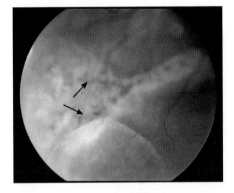

Figure 10-20   Rhegmatogenous RD, chronic   *Chronic RD (*right *of arrows) with pigmented demarcation line* (arrows).

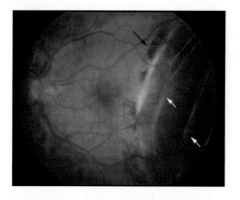

Figure 10-21 Rhegmatogenous RD, chronic *Chronic RD* (black arrow) *with multiple demarcation lines and some subretinal fibrous bands* (white arrows).

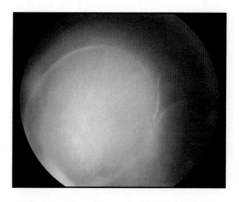

Figure 10-22 Rhegmatogenous RD, chronic *Retinal cysts associated with chronic RD.*

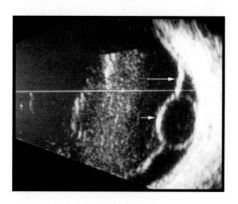

Figure 10-23 Rhegmatogenous RD, chronic *B-scan ultrasound of retinal cyst* (short arrow) *and chronic RD* (long arrow).

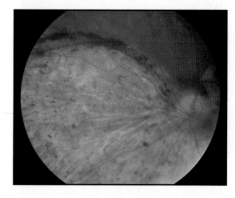

Figure 10-24 Rhegmatogenous RD, regressed *Pigmentation from spontaneously regressed RD.*

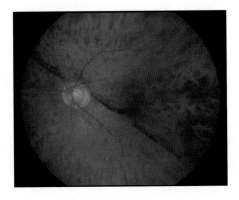

Figure 10-25 Rhegmatogenous RD, pigmentary disturbances *Subretinal dispersion of pigment after repair of "macula-off" RD.*

Visual potential is directly related to presence and duration of macular involvement (Figure 10-25). Retinal detachments not involving the macula often recover vision fully. "Macula-off" RDs usually lead to permanent reduction of central vision even when repaired properly. Recovery often takes months, and the degree of recovery diminishes with longer periods of macular detachment.

Treatment Options

LASER PHOTOCOAGULATION Used alone it has a limited role in management of RD. Usually it cannot seal a retinal break closed in the presence of subretinal fluid. Laser treatment may be used to create a barrier ("wall off the detachment") to prevent progression of the detachment. It is especially useful in chronic inferior retinal detachment or in cases where systemic illness prevents more definitive repair.

CRYOTHERAPY (See preceding discussion of "Laser Photocoagulation.") Occasionally RDs with very shallow fluid around the retinal break can be cured by treating the break with cryotherapy alone.

PNEUMATIC RETINOPEXY An intravitreal gas bubble is used to tamponade the retinal break closed temporarily. The subretinal fluid will resolve and either laser photocoagulation or cryotherapy is used to permanently close the retinal break(s). The success rate is high and varies with patient selection. Patients with phakic RDs with a single, superior retinal break without vitreous hemorrhage, extensive lattice degeneration, or early proliferative vitreoretinopathy (PVR) do best. This relatively noninvasive, low-cost, quick-recovery office procedure is gaining in acceptance.

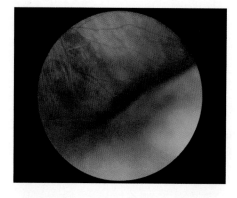

Figure 10-26 Rhegmatogenous RD, subretinal hemorrhage *Subretinal hemorrhage beneath the attached retina associated with drainage of subretinal fluid during scleral buckling surgery.*

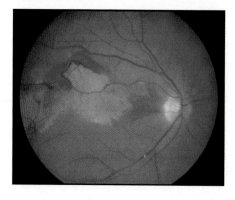

Figure 10-27 Rhegmatogenous RD, subretinal hemorrhage *Macular extension of subretinal blood complicating drainage of subretinal fluid.*

TEMPORARY BALLOON   This treatment consists of an external device applied via small conjunctival incisions. The balloon temporarily indents the sclera to allow cryotherapy or a laser-induced chorioretinal adhesion to form. This treatment option is especially useful for inferior RD when pneumatic retinopexy is not an option; however, it is not a widely used technique.

SCLERAL BUCKLE   This widely applied technique consists of indentation of the sclera using a flexible silicone sponge or strip that is permanently sutured on or within the sclera to relieve vitreoretinal traction on the retinal break(s).

Cryotherapy is generally used to create permanent adhesion although postoperative laser therapy can be applied. Drainage of subretinal fluid or injection of intravitreal gas, or both, are also sometimes performed to assist in reattachment. Success rates of over 95% have been reported for repair of primary RD.

Side effects and complications of the scleral buckle include:

Pain
Infection
Hemorrhage (especially with drainage of subretinal fluid; Figures 10-26 and 10-27)

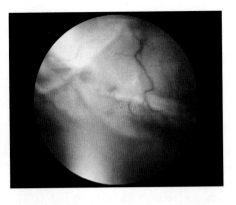

Figure 10-28   Rhegmatogenous RD, retinal incarceration   *Incarceration of the retina into the drainage site during scleral buckle.*

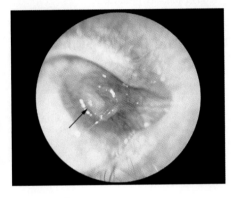

Figure 10-29   Scleral buckle   *Extruding scleral buckle* (arrow).

Retinal incarceration at drainage site (Figure 10-28)
Induced myopia
Diplopia
Extrusion or intrusion (Figure 10-29)
Anterior segment ischemia
Ptosis

VITRECTOMY   This technique is increasingly used in managing primary RD with or without a scleral buckle. It allows for direct release of vitreoretinal traction. Intravitreal gas or silicone oil is used to tamponade the retina while retinopexy with laser or cryotherapy takes effect.

Vitrectomy is especially useful for RDs with posterior breaks, PVR, vitreous hemorrhage, or a tight orbit preventing scleral buckle.

Side effects and complications of vitrectomy include

Elevated intraocular pressure
Cataract
Dislocation of intraocular lens
Infection
Hemorrhage
Postoperative positioning (e.g., face-down) may be needed

PROLIFERATIVE VITREORETINOPATHY

Definition

Proliferative vitreoretinopathy (PVR) refers to the development of preretinal, subretinal, and even intraretinal fibrous proliferation that induces traction and distortion of the retina in the presence of RD (Table 10-1).

Epidemiology and Etiology

In the presence of RD, activation of vitreous glial cells and metaplasia of retinal pigment epithelial cells produces fibrous tissue that proliferates on and under the retina. Although the mechanism is not totally understood, risk factors include RDs with multiple retinal breaks, large retinal breaks, chronicity, vitreous hemorrhage, and trauma. Proliferative vitreoretinopathy may be primary or develop after attempted repair of RD. It tends to occur 3 weeks to 3 months after initial repair.

History

The same as for RD.

Important Clinical Signs

The retina is relatively immobile with fixed folds. Rolled edges of the retinal break(s) and extensive pigment in vitreous, on and under retina are noted (Figures 10-30 and 10-31). Vitreous bands are prominent.

Associated Clinical Signs

Hypotony
Anterior flare or uveitis
Rubeosis iridis

TABLE 10-1   CLASSIFICATION OF PROLIFERATIVE VITREORETINOPATHY

Grade A	Vitreous haze, vitreous pigment clumps, and pigment clusters inferior to retina
Grade B	Inner retinal wrinkling, retinal stiffness, vessel tortuosity, rolled edge of break, and decreased vitreous mobility
Grade C	P (posterior)—expressed in the number (1–12) clock hours involvement
	Focal, diffuse, or circumferential full-thickness folds, subretinal strands
	A (anterior)—expressed in the number (1–12) clock hours involvement
	Focal, diffuse, or circumferential full-thickness folds; subretinal strands; condensed vitreous; and anterior displacement of vitreous base with anterior trough.

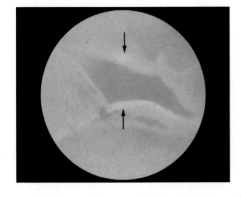

Figure 10-30   Proliferative vitreo-retinopathy (PVR), retinal edge rolled
Rolled edge of a retinal tear (arrows) *indicating early PVR.*

Differential Diagnosis

Purely tractional RD (e.g., diabetic retinopathy; Figure 10-32A)

Exudative RD

Diagnostic Evaluation

Diagnosis is based on indirect ophthalmoscopy. Ultrasound may show the rigid nature of RD if detachment cannot be directly visualized.

Prognosis and Management

Proliferative vitreoretinopathy almost always progresses, causing severe visual loss. Repair is difficult, especially for more advanced degrees of PVR (see Table 10-1). Repair almost always includes vitrectomy, often with a high encircling scleral buckle as well as a long-lasting vitreous gas or silicone oil tamponade. Recurrence rate is high, and recovery of excellent visual acuity is uncommon in severe cases (Figures 10-32B and 10-33A,B).

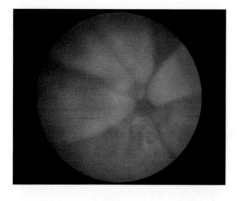

Figure 10-31   PVR, fixed retinal folds
Severe PVR in a napkin-ring configuration with fixed retinal folds.

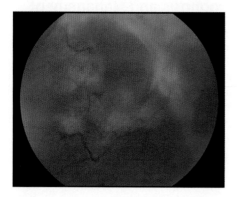

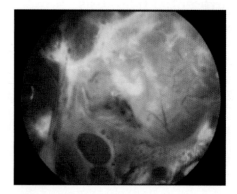

Figure 10-32A   Tractional RD associated with proliferative diabetic retinopathy
Fibrovascular proliferation is extending from the optic disc along the retinal vascular arcades, elevating the retina in a "wolf-jaw" configuration.

Figure 10-32B   PVR, recurrent RD
Recurrent RD with severe PVR. Note severe fibrous proliferation on the retinal surface and associated retinal breaks.

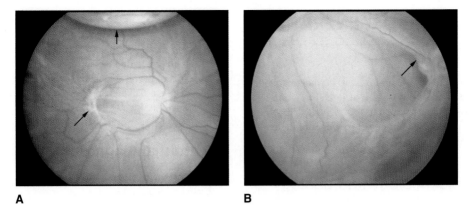

Figure 10-33   PVR, fixed retinal folds   *A. PVR with macular pucker* (long arrow) *after vitrectomy and scleral buckle for RD. Note the edge of the slowly clearing vitreous gas bubble* (short arrow) *used during the initial repair.* **B.** *Inferior proliferation causing tractional elevation of the retina* (arrow).

LATTICE DEGENERATION

Definition

Lattice degeneration is a peripheral fundus abnormality consisting of retinal thinning with loss of inner retinal tissue and unusually strong vitreoretinal adhesion at the edges of the retinal excavation.

Epidemiology and Etiology

The condition is common, occurring in about 8% of the population. It is more common and more extensive in patients with myopia.

History

Patients are asymptomatic except when the condition is associated with retinal tear and detachment formation.

Important Clinical Signs

Lattice degeneration can be variable in pigmentation, circumferential extent, and orientation (usually concentric with ora serrata but may be radial or perivascular) (Figure 10-34). Cross-hatched white lines, which give the appearance of a lattice, are often not present. Indirect ophthalmoscopy is usually necessary to see lattice degeneration. Dynamic scleral depression is the key to appreciating the inner retinal excavation.

Associated Clinical Signs

Myopia.
Stickler's syndrome—This syndrome, which has an autosomal-dominant inheritance, consists of vitreoretinopathy with arthropathy and other systemic features.

Retinal breaks—atrophic round holes are often present within the lattice degeneration, sometimes with associated subretinal fluid. Tractional flap tears may occur, usually at the edges of the lattice (Figure 10-35).

Differential Diagnosis

Cobblestone degeneration
Cystoid degeneration
Retinoschisis
Vitreoretinal tuft
Pigmented or atrophic chorioretinal scars
Grouped pigmentation

Diagnostic Evaluation

Indirect ophthalmoscopy is performed with scleral depression. Peripheral contact lens examination may help confirm the presence of associated tears.

Prognosis and Management

Usually this condition is of no clinical significance. The risk of RD increases with the extent of lattice degeneration. Prophylactic treatment (laser or cryotherapy) generally is not indicated except if the fellow eye had lattice-related RD. A strong family history of retinal tear or RD or anticipated intraocular surgery are other possible considerations for treatment.

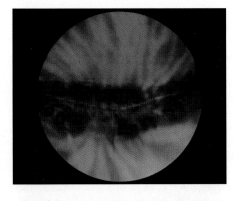

Figure 10-34   Pigmented lattice degeneration   *Note the lattice-like network within the area of increased pigmentation.*

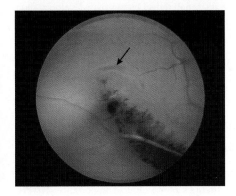

Figure 10-35   Lattice degeneration with associated horseshoe tear and RD (arrow)
A horseshoe tear at the edge of lattice reflects firm vitreoretinal adhesion at the edge of the lattice degeneration.

VITREORETINAL TUFT AND MERIDIONAL FOLD

Definition

Vitreoretinal tuft and meridional fold are common structural abnormalities of the extreme retinal periphery with unusually strong vitreoretinal adhesion. They are infrequently the cause of rhegmatogenous RD.

Epidemiology and Etiology

Vitreoretinal tufts are very common in the general population and are the source of RD in less than 1% of all affected patients. Meridional folds are very common in the general population and are the source of RD in less than 1% of all affected patients. They are a developmental abnormality.

History

The abnormalities are asymptomatic except when they precipitate RD.

Important Clinical Signs

Vitreoretinal tufts are small areas of substantial focal vitreous traction producing a discrete retinal elevation (Figure 10-36). There may be pigment around the tuft. They often are mistaken for small flap tears, but no full-thickness break is present.

Meridional folds are folds of redundant retina (Figure 10-37). Most often superonasal, they may straddle and are perpendicular to the ora serrata. Small retinal breaks may develop at their posterior end.

Differential Diagnosis

Retinal tear
"Snowball" or other inflammatory precipitate

Prognosis and Management

Both abnormalities are almost always incidental findings of no clinical importance. Rarely, they may be the only abnormal finding in cases of RD and are presumed to be the cause of the detachment. They are generally treated with cryotherapy or laser photocoagulation at the time of RD repair, but prophylactic treatment is not warranted.

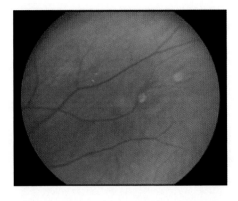

Figure 10-36   Vitreoretinal tuft   *Focal opacification and elevation of the retina occurs at two grey-white vitreoretinal tufts.*

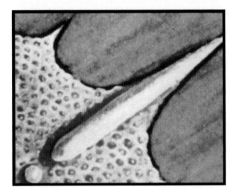

Figure 10-37   Schematic of meridional fold   *The fold represents a pleat of retina between the ora bays.*

COBBLESTONE DEGENERATION

Definition

Cobblestone degeneration describes discrete circular areas of peripheral atrophy of the retina, RPE, and choriocapillaris.

Synonym—paving stone degeneration.

Epidemiology and Etiology

This is a degenerative process of unknown etiology. The condition is more common in the elderly.

History

Patients are usually asymptomatic.

Important Clinical Signs

Circular areas of thinning of the retina with depigmentation are seen (Figure 10-38). Often a pigmented halo is noted. The degeneration is most common inferiorly and is usually bilateral.

Differential Diagnosis

Retinal breaks
Lattice degeneration
Congenital hypertrophy of RPE

Diagnostic Evaluation

Diagnosis is based on indirect ophthalmoscopy.

Prognosis and Management

Cobblestone degeneration is of no clinical importance. It is not a predisposing condition for RD and, in fact, may be protective against a progressive RD.

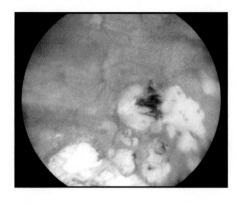

Figure 10-38   Cobblestone (paving stone) degeneration   *Areas of pigmentation are observed within the discrete areas of depigmentation.*

PERIPHERAL GROUPED PIGMENTATION

Definition

Peripheral grouped pigmentation describes a cluster of flat, discrete pigmented spots deep to retina.

Epidemiology and Etiology

It may occur at any age, in both genders. This is a congenital abnormality.

History

Patients are usually asymptomatic.

Important Clinical Signs

A cluster of flat, uniformly pigmented spots of variable size are often noted (Figure 10-39). These are also known as "bear tracks" because of their paw-print appearance. Rarely, the pigmentation is bilateral.

Associated Clinical Signs

There are no signs of inflammation, fluid, or elevation.

Differential Diagnosis

Cobblestone degeneration
Choroidal nevus or melanoma
Lattice degeneration
Chorioretinal scar

Important: Peripheral grouped pigmentation must be distinguished from the pigmented spots in the fundus that are seen in familial polyposis (Gardner's syndrome). This autosomal-dominant condition, which is usually asymptomatic, often includes flat, variably pigmented spots in the fundus. Lesions of Gardner's syndrome tend to be more oval, with an irregularly pigmented "comet's tail" (Figure 10-40). Affected patients have a very high risk of colonic carcinoma. Fundus lesions in Gardner's syndrome are usually seen as early as infancy. For patients with a positive family history, the presence of fundus lesions is virtually diagnostic of the systemic syndrome.

Diagnostic Evaluation

Diagnosis is based on indirect ophthalmoscopy. For suspicious lesions (see preceding discussion), obtain a family history of gastrointestinal malignancy and consider colonoscopy.

Prognosis and Management

Peripheral grouped pigmentation is of no clinical importance with no potential for RD or malignant transformation.

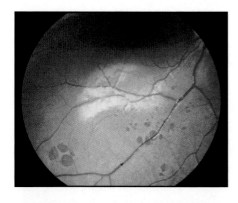

Figure 10-39   Grouped pigmentation
Small clumps of grouped pigmentation ("bear tracks," inset) *have little risk of malignant transformation.*

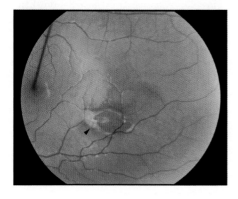

Figure 10-40   Pigmented fundus lesions associated with Gardner's syndrome
Note the depigmented halo (arrowhead) *and oblong shape of the lesion.*

DEGENERATIVE RETINOSCHISIS

Definition

Degenerative retinoschisis is a splitting of the retina that produces elevation of the inner retina, mimicking a detachment.

Epidemiology and Etiology

The condition is a degenerative process that begins with peripheral cystoid degeneration. Further splitting in the outer plexiform layer leads to the elevation noted clinically. Degenerative retinoschisis affects both genders and all races.

History

Patients are asymptomatic except in rare cases of progressive retinal detachment.

Important Clinical Signs

A transparent dome-shaped elevation of peripheral retina may be easily overlooked (Figures 10-41 and 10-42). A thin, cystic appearance is noted. The inferotemporal fundus is most often affected. In the majority of cases the condition is bilateral. The retina is immobile, and there is no associated pigmentation of the RPE or vitreous.

Associated Clinical Signs

White "snowflakes" on the underside of the inner retinal layer or a pockmarked appearance may be noted. Outer wall holes are circular, and there are sometimes multiple defects (Figure 10-43). Detection of an intact, overlying, inner layer is facilitated by noting retinal vessels coursing over the hole. An absolute visual field defect corresponds to the area of retinoschisis.

Differential Diagnosis

Rhegmatogenous RD—the presence of a retinal break, corrugations, undulations, pigment in vitreous or demarcation lines, symptoms, hypotony, and a fellow eye that is normal help distinguish this condition from retinoschisis.

Exudative retinal detachment—associated tumor or inflammatory signs, shifting fluid, and symptoms suggest this etiology.

Juvenile retinoschisis (X-linked)—this heritable condition produces a stellate foveal appearance with splitting neurosensory retina within the nerve fiber layer. It may present as vitreous hemorrhage.

Diagnostic Evaluation

Evaluation consists of indirect ophthalmoscopy with scleral depression and contact lens examination. The fellow eye should also be examined.

Prognosis and Management

Degenerative retinoschisis rarely produces vision loss. Progression to posterior retina or development of true rhegmatogenous detachment is uncommon. Outer wall defects usually are easily detected, but inner wall breaks are difficult to identify. In cases of very posterior retinoschisis with progression, outer wall breaks may be surrounded with laser treatment (Figure 10-44). If the outer layer is detached as well, then surgery, usually vitrectomy, is needed.

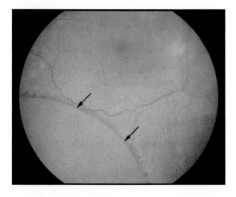

Figure 10-41 Peripheral retinoschisis
*Note the smooth, dome-shaped elevation in
the inferotemporal quadrant* (arrows).

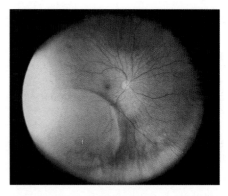

Figure 10-42 Degenerative retinoschisis
*Wide-angle photograph of inferotemporal
retinoschisis* (lower left). *The external
transillumination is noted* (directly left).

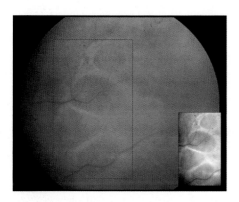

**Figure 10-43 Degenerative retinoschisis,
outer wall breaks** *Outer wall holes
associated with retinoschisis* (inset) *are
required to cause a retinoschisis-associated
retinal detachment. Note that the inner-layer
retinal vessels course over the outer-layer
retinal holes.*

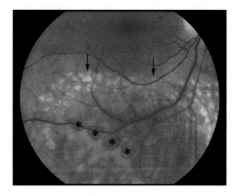

**Figure 10-44 Degenerative retinoschisis,
outer wall breaks** *Laser treatment*
(arrows) *surrounding outer wall holes*
(asterisks) *in retinoschisis.*

EXUDATIVE RETINAL DETACHMENT

Definition

Exudative retinal detachment describes elevation of the retina by fluid that leaks from within or under the retina.

Epidemiology and Etiology

By definition, the retinal elevation is not due to a retinal break. Breakdown of the normal inner (retinal vascular endothelial cells) or outer blood-retinal barrier (RPE) produces exudation of fluid, elevating the retina. Cases can be divided into one of four categories, as follows:

Inflammatory

Scleritis
Harada's disease
Sympathetic ophthalmia
Orbital pseudotumor and other orbital inflammation
Infectious retinochoroidis (e.g., toxoplasmosis, syphilis, Lyme disease, bartonellosis)
Vasculitis or autoimmune (e.g., lupus, polyarteritis nodosa)

Vascular

Coats' disease (Figure 10-45)
Retinal capillary hemangioma
Acute systemic hypertension
Eclampsia
Disseminated intravascular coagulation (DIC)
Renal failure

Neoplastic

Choroidal melanoma (Figure 10-46)
Choroidal metastasis
Retinoblastoma

Miscellaneous

Bullous central serous choroidopathy
Uveal effusion syndrome
Nanophthalmos
Coloboma

History

Patients experience a progressive, often fluctuating loss of peripheral vision, that is similar to rhegmatogenous RD, but often more variable in course. Visual changes may be positional, caused by shifting subretinal fluid with changes in head position. If inflammatory in nature, the condition may cause pain; however, it is often asymptomatic.

Important Clinical Signs

There is a dome-shaped elevation of the retina, which retains its transparency (Figure 10-47). The subretinal fluid generally shifts to the most gravity-dependent position with changes in the patient's head position.

Associated Clinical Signs

Observe for features of the underlying cause, such as inflammation, vascular changes, or solid tumor (see Figure 10-46).

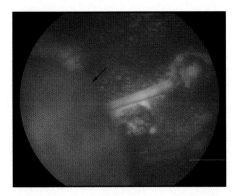

Figure 10-45 Exudative RD associated with Coats' disease (arrow) *Note the sub-retinal lipid precipitates where the exudative RD is shallower.*

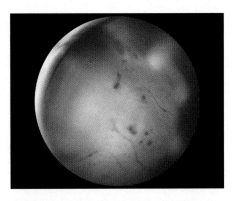

Figure 10-46 Exudative RD overlying choroidal melanoma with retinal hemorrhages *This smooth, domed-shaped elevation extends beyond the choroidal melanoma.*

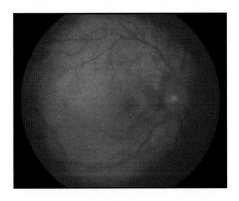

Figure 10-47 Exudative RD *This detachment exhibited shifting subretinal fluid with change of position.*

Differential Diagnosis

Rhegmatogenous RD (especially chronic with small retinal break)

Retinoschisis

Choroidal detachment

Diagnostic Evaluation

Fluorescein angiography—often shows source(s) of subretinal fluid and the nature of the defect causing it (see discussion under "Epidemiology and Etiology," earlier).

B-scan ultrasound—thickening of sclera is seen in scleritis or orbital inflammation. Calcification suggests retinoblastoma. Identify features of choroidal tumor or thickening.

A-scan ultrasound—short axial length is typical of nanophthalmos.

Prognosis and Management

The prognosis varies markedly, depending on the underlying etiology. Treatment depends on the underlying cause.

CHOROIDAL DETACHMENT

Definition

Choroidal detachment refers to elevation of the retina and choroid by either accumulation of serous fluid or blood in the suprachoroidal space.

Epidemiology and Etiology

Serous choroidal detachment is generally a secondary effect of another underlying problem. Causes include:

Hypotony
Wound leak
Postglaucoma surgery
Cyclodialysis cleft
Inflammation
High scleral buckle

Hemorrhagic choroidal detachment may occur spontaneously, intraoperatively after trauma, or as the result of vascular abnormalities such as choroidal neovascularization.

History

Occurrence of a visual field defect or shadow may be gradual or sudden in onset. There may be associated severe pain, if hemorrhagic.

Important Clinical Signs

A dome-shaped elevation of the retina and choroid is noted. The retina and choroid may appear normal in every way except for their relative position within the eye. If large enough, the detachment may obstruct the examiner's view of the optic nerve and macula. If elevations are very large, they may contact each other in vitreous cavity ("kissing choroidals").

Associated Clinical Signs

Hypotony
Marked elevation of intraocular pressure (hemorrhagic choroidals)
Vitreous hemorrhage
Retinal folds or detachment
Shallow anterior chamber

Differential Diagnosis

Choroidal melanoma
Choroidal metastasis
Retinal detachment
Retinoschisis
Scleral buckle

Diagnostic Evaluation

If choroidal detachment is associated with hypotony, look for the cause (e.g., gonioscopy for cyclodialysis cleft). B-scan ultrasonography confirms the diagnosis and helps distinguish between serous and hemorrhagic detachment. It also will show evidence of inflammation of the sclera or orbit, and can help distinguish detachment from neoplasm.

Prognosis and Management

The prognosis for patients with serous choroidal detachment is generally favorable if the underlying etiology can be reversed. Restoration of normal intraocular pressure and eradication of inflammation are generally adequate to reverse this process. Hemorrhagic detachment can produce severe pain or marked elevation of intraocular pressure requiring prompt surgical drainage. Otherwise, the condition can generally be observed and will slowly resolve. If the vitreous or retina are adherent to anterior structures such as a cataract wound, then vitrectomy is indicated or else retinal detachment will occur as the choroidal detachment resolves. Surgical drainage is usually recommended for "kissing choroidals," although the necessity and optimal timing of this procedure are controversial.

Appendix A
TABLES

TABLE A-1   **LEUKOKORIA**

Congenital cataract
PFVS (persistent fetal vasculature), also called PHPV (persistent hyperplastic primary vitreous)
Retinopathy of prematurity
Retinoblastoma
Medulloblastoma
Retinal dysplasia
Coats' disease
Large chorioretinal coloboma
Long-standing retinal detachment
Intraocular inflammation
Medulloepithelioma
Norrie's disease
Incontinentia pigmenti

TABLE A-2 RETINAL VASCULITIS

Retinal Phlebitis
Sarcoidosis
Tuberculosis
Syphilis
Multiple sclerosis
Pars planitis
Eales' disease
Antiphospholipid antibody syndrome
HIV
Frosted branch angiitis

Retinal Arteritis
Behçhet's disease
Polyarteritis nodosa
Collagen vascular disease
Associated vasculitis
Toxoplasmosis
Eales' disease
HIV
Antiphospholipid antibody syndrome
Syphilis

HIV = human immunodeficiency virus.

TABLE A-3 PSEUDOCYSTOID MACULAR EDEMA

Juvenile X-linked retinoschisis
Retinitis pigmentosa
Nicotinic acid use
Goldmann-Favre disease

TABLE A-4 FOVEAL HYPOPLASIA

Albinism
Aniridia
PHPV (persistent hyperplastic primary vitreous) (see Table A-1)
Achromatopsia

TABLE A-5 CHOROIDAL FOLDS

Choroidal mass
Hypotony
Hyperthyroidism
Hyperopia
Postoperative
Retinal detachment repair
Orbital mass
Inflammation
Disciform scar

TABLE A-6 CHOROIDAL DETACHMENT AFTER CATARACT SURGERY

Wound leak
Cyclodialysis cleft
Retinal detachment
Uveitis
Inadvertent perforation of the globe

TABLE A-7 CLASSIC MASQUERADERS

I. Anterior Segment Pathology

1. Retinoblastoma	Pseudohypopyon, anterior chamber cell and flare
2. Leukemia	Iris heterochromia, anterior chamber cell and flare
3. Intraocular foreign body (IOFB)	Anterior chamber cell and flare, metals may pigment uveal tissue, chronic uveitis
4. Malignant melanoma	Anterior chamber cell and flare, glaucoma
5. Juvenile xanthogranuloma	Spontaneous hyphema, anterior chamber cell and flare

II. Posterior Segment Pathology

1. Lymphoma (formerly called reticulum cell sarcoma)	Vitreous cells, retinal hemorrhage and exudates, retinal pigment epithelial infiltrates
2. Retinoblastoma	Vitreous cells, diffuse uveitis, retinal exudates, rubeosis iridis
3. Malignant melanoma	Vitreous cells, angle-closure glaucoma
4. Submacular hemorrhage	Choroidal malignant melanoma
5. Peripheral retinal detachment	Anterior chamber cell and flare, uveitic glaucoma
6. HIV (human immunodeficiency virus)	Cotton-wool spots, retinal microangiopathy, hypertensive retinopathy, cystoid macular edema
7. Spirochetes (Lyme disease, syphilis)	Cystoid macular edema, uveitis, papillitis
9. Retained IOFB	Chronic uveitis, vitritis of unknown etiology
10. Central serous retinopathy	Circumscribed choroidal hemangioma (serous macular detachment)
11. Posterior scleritis	Choroidal mass, angle-closure glaucoma
12. Polypoidal choroidal vasculopathy	Exudative age-related macular degeneration
13. Cystoid macular edema	Choroidal neovascularization

TABLE A-8   LASER PHOTOCOAGULATION TREATMENT GUIDELINES

I. Focal Laser for Diabetic Macular Edema

A. *Duration:* 0.1 sec

B. *Spot Size:* 50–100 μm

C. *Power:* 100 mW and increase by 20–30 mW as needed

D. *Wavelength:* Green or yellow

E. *Technique:* Light- (grey) to medium- (grey-white) intensity spots directed at leaking microaneurysms in areas of retinal thickening. No spots within 500 μm of foveal center with first treatment and within 300 μm with subsequent treatments. Avoid treating intraretinal hemorrhage (macular pucker).

II. Grid Laser for Diffuse Macular Edema (Diabetes or Branch Vein Occlusions)

A. *Duration:* 0.1 sec

B. *Spot Size:* 100 μm

C. *Power:* 100 mW and increase by 20–30 mW as needed

D. *Wavelength:* Green or yellow

E. *Technique:* Light- to medium-intensity spots placed in a grid fashion 1 spot width apart being directed to areas of retinal thickening associated with either diffuse leakage or capillary nonperfusion on FA. No spots within 500 μm of foveal center. Avoid intraretinal hemorrhage.

III. Focal Laser for Choroidal Neovascularization

A. *Duration:* 0.2–0.5 sec or longer

B. *Spot Size:* 200 μm

C. *Power:* 200 mW and increase by 50 mW as needed

D. *Wavelength:* Green, yellow, or red (depending on proximity to foveola)

E. *Technique:* High-intensity, overlapping, confluent spots completely covering entire choroidal neovascular complex (as guided by FA) with minimum of 100-μm margin. Treat over thin, adjacent subretinal blood.

IV. Scatter Laser for Disc, Retinal, or Iris Neovascularization

A. *Duration:* 0.1–0.2 sec

B. *Spot Size:* 200–500 μm (adjust for magnifying effects of panfunduscopic lenses)

C. *Power:* 200 mW and increase by 50 mW as needed

D. *Wavelength:* Green, yellow, or red (depending on media opacities)

E. *Technique:* Medium-intensity spots, one-half to one spot width apart.

   1. Initial treatment: Start with applications about ½ to 1 disc diameter anterior to disc and temporal arcades and greater than 2 disc diameters temporal to fovea. Laser spots should extend out to the equator.

   2. For proliferative diabetic retinopathy and central retinal vein occlusions: Panretinal scatter (i.e., 360 degrees) will be needed, applying about 1600–3000 spots to start with over two or three sessions and adding as needed thereafter.

   3. For branch retinal vein occlusions: Spots are applied in sector of involvement and can be placed in one session. Avoid intraretinal hemorrhage and major retinal vessels.

FA = Fluorescein angiography.

TABLE A-9   CHOROIDAL NEOVASCULARIZATION AND ASSOCIATED CONDITIONS

CNV in Patients > 50 Years
  Age-related macular degeneration

CNV in Patients < 50 Years
  Pathologic myopia
  Presumed ocular histoplasmosis syndrome
  Idiopathic CNV of the young
  Angioid streaks

Others Conditions Associated with CNV
  Hereditary/Congenital
    Best's vitelliform dystrophy
    Sorsby's macular dystrophy
    Adult foveomacular dystrophy
    Choroideremia
    Coloboma (chorioretinal, retinal)
    Fundus flavimaculatus (Stargardt's disease)
    Osteogenesis imperfecta
    Retinitis pigmentosa
    Dominant drusen
    Optic nerve pit
  Inflammatory/Infections
    Acute posterior multifocal placoid pigment epitheliopathy (APMPPE)
    Birdshot choroidopathy
    Recurrent multifocal choroiditis (punctate inner choroiditis, multifocal choroiditis)
    Rubella
    Fungal chorioretinitis (*Candida, Aspergillus,* others)
    Sarcoidosis
    Serpiginous (choroiditis geographic helicoid peripapillary choroiditis)
    Toxoplasmosis
    Vogt-Koyanagi-Harada syndrome
    Sympathetic ophthalmia
    Toxocara canis
    Syphilis
  Traumatic
    Laser photocoagulation
    Choroidal rupture
    Intraocular foreign body
    Subretinal fluid drainage (internal, external)
    Scleral perforation
  Tumor
    Choroidal nevus
    Choroidal osteoma
    Combined retinal–retinal pigment epithelial hamartoma
    Choroidal melanoma
    Choroidal hemangioma
    Metastatic carcinoma
  Other
    Chronic retinal detachment   Drusen (optic nerve head)
    Central serous retinopathy   Macular hole
    Decompensated retinal pigment epitheliopathy   Retinal telangiectasis
    Neovascularization of the ora serrata

CNV = choroidal neovascularization.

TABLE A-10 DIFFERENTIAL DIAGNOSIS OF A CHOROIDAL MASS ("PSEUDOMELANOMA")

Condition	Key Differentiating Features	Diagnostic Test(s)
Lesions Involving the Retina		
Retinal cavernous hemangioma	Multilobular contour	IVFA
Astrocytic hamartoma	Superficial location; pale color; calcifications; association with tuberous sclerosis	IVFA, ultrasonography
Lesions Involving the RPE		
Combined hamartoma of the retina and RPE	Overlying fibroglial tissue; distortion of retinal vessels	IVFA
Congenital hypertrophy of the RPE	Flat; well-demarcated; marginal halo	IVFA
Reactive hyperplasia of the RPE	History of inflammation or trauma; dark black; often multifocal	
Disciform scar of age-related macular degeneration	Bilaterality; macular drusen; peripheral RPE changes	IVFA
Adenoma of the RPE	Black color; abruptly elevated margin; propensity for vitreous hemorrhage	

Condition	Key Differentiating Features	Diagnostic Test(s)
Lesions Involving the Choroid		
Choroidal nevus	Surface drusen	Serial fundus photographs
Choroidal melanoma	Growth; orange pigment; predilection for whites	Serial photographs and ultrasonography
Metastatic carcinoma	Medical history; less elevated; hypopigmentation	Fine-needle aspiration biopsy
Circumscribed choroidal hemangioma	Orange-red or yellow in color	IVFA, ICGA, ultrasonography
Choroidal osteoma	Posterior location; yellow color; predilection for young women	Ultrasonography, computed tomography
Melanocytoma	Dark black color; feathered margins	Serial fundus photographs
Inflammatory Conditions		
Choroidal granuloma	Inflammation; lack of pigment; medical history	Careful review of systems; testing for sarcoidosis, syphilis, tuberculosis
Posterior scleritis	Inflammation; choroidal folds; responsive to corticosteroids	Ultrasonography
Choroidal detachment	History of ocular trauma or surgery	

ICGA = indocyanine green angiography;
IVFA = intravenous fluorescein angiography;
RPE = retinal pigment epithelium.

TABLE A-11 RETINAL DISEASES WITH IDENTIFIED GENETIC DEFECTS

	Mode of Transmission	Disease Locus	Gene	Gene Product or Function
Diseases Principally Affecting the Outer Retina				
Retinitis pigmentosa	AD	3q21-q24	rhodopsin	Signal transduction
		6p21.2-cen	peripherin/RDS	Peripherin/RDS
		8q11-q13	RP1	Unknown function
		11q13	ROM1	Retinal outer segment membrane protein 1
		14q11.2	NRL	Retinal transcription factor
	AR	1p31	RPE65	Unknown function
		2q14.1	MERTK	c-mer Receptor tyrosine kinase
		4p16.3	PDE6B	Rod cGMP phosphodiesterase beta subunit
		4p12-cen	CNGA1	Rod cGMP-gated channel, alpha subunit
		5q31.2-q34	PDE6A	cGMP phosphodiesterase alpha subunit
		6p21.3	TULP1	Photoreceptor protein
		8q13.1-13.3	TTPA	Alpha tocopherol transfer protein
		10q23	RGR	RPE-retinal G protein–coupled receptor
		15q26	RLBP1	Cellular retinaldehyde-binding protein
	X-linked	Xp21.1	RPGR	Unknown function
		Xp11.3	RP2	Similar to human cofactor C
Congenital stationary night blindness	AD	3p22	GNAT1	Rod transducin alpha subunit
		3q21-q24	rhodopsin	Signal transduction
		4p16.3	PDE6B	Rod cGMP phosphodiesterase beta subunit
Oguchi type	AR	2q37.1	arrestin	Phototransduction
		13q34	RHOK	Rhodopsin kinase
	X-linked	Xp11.4	nyctalopin	Extracellular proteoglycan
		Xp11.23	CACNA1F	Voltage-gated calcium channel, alpha-1 subunit
Cone dystrophy	AD	6p21.1	GUCA1A	Guanylate cyclase activating protein 1A
Cone-rod dystrophy	AD	17p13.1	GUCY2D	Retina-specific guanylate cyclase

Disease	Inheritance	Locus	Gene	Protein function
		17q11.2	UNC119	Unknown function
		19q13.3	CRX	Photoreceptor transcription factor
Achromatopsia	AR	2q11	CNGA3	Cone cGMP-gated cation channel, alpha subunit
Enhanced S-cone syndrome	AR	15q23	NR2E3	Nuclear receptor subfamily 2 group E3

Diseases Principally Affecting the RPE and Choroid

Diffuse Dystrophies

Disease	Inheritance	Locus	Gene	Protein function
Stargardt's disease	AD	6q14	ELOVL4	Elongation of very long fatty acids protein
	AR	1p21-p22	ABCA4	ATP-binding cassette transporter
Fundus albipunctatus	AR	12q13-q14	RDH5	11-cis Retinol dehydrogenase 5
Choroideremia	X-linked	Xq21.1-q21.3	CHM	rab Geranylgeranyl transferase escort protein
Gyrate atrophy	AR	10q26	OAT	Omithine aminotransferase
RPE degeneration	AR	10q24	RBP4	Retinol-binding protein 4
Leber's congenital amaurosis	AR	1p31	RPE65	Unknown function
		14q11	RPGRIP-1	Unknown function
		17p13.1	GUCY2D	Retinal-specific guanylate cyclase
		17p13.1	AIPL1	? Nuclear transport

Macular Dystrophies

Disease	Inheritance	Locus	Gene	Protein function
Sorsby macular dystrophy	AD	22q12.1-q13.2	TIMP-3	Tissue inhibitor of metalloproteinases-3
Best's vitelliform dystrophy	AD	11q13	bestrophin	? Fatty acid transport
Malattia levitenense (Doyne honeycomb dystrophy)	AD	2p16-p21	EFEMP1	Fibrillin-like extracellular matrix protein-1

Diseases Principally Affecting Inner Retina/Vitreoretinal Interface

Disease	Inheritance	Locus	Gene	Protein function
Familial exudative vitreoretinopathy	X-linked	Xp11.3	NDP	Unknown function
Norrie's disease	X-linked	Xp11.3	NDP	Unknown function
Retinoschisis	X-linked	Xp22.2	retinoschisin	Photoreceptor-specific

AD = autosomal dominant; AR = autosomal recessive; ATP = adenosine triphosphate; cGMP = cyclic guanosine monophosphate; RPE = retinal pigment epithelium.

INDEX

Note: Page numbers followed by *f* or *t* indicate figures and tables, respectively.

Gass classification, of idiopathic macular hole, 26, 26t
Genetic counseling, retinoblastoma and, 183
Genetic defects, retinal diseases associated with, 296t–297t
Geographic atrophy, in dry age-related macular degeneration, 3, 4, 4f
Giant tear of retina, 259, 260f
Glaucoma, and nonproliferative diabetic retinopathy, 58
Goldmann perimetry, for retinitis pigmentosa, 171
Granuloma, choroidal, 295t
Grid laser photocoagulation, for branch retinal vein obstruction, 97
Grönblad-Strandberg syndrome, and angioid streaks, 40, 40t
Gyrate atrophy, 156, 160–161, 161f, 297t

HAART. See Highly active antiretroviral therapy
Haemophilus influenzae, and bleb-associated endophthalmitis, 116
Hagberg-Santavuori disease, 174
Hamartoma
   astrocytic, 178–179, 179f, 295t
   of retina and retinal pigment epithelium, 190, 191f, 295f
Hard drusen. See Small drusen
Hard yellow exudates (HYE), in nonproliferative diabetic retinopathy, 57f, 58f, 62t
Hemangioma
   choroidal, 200–201, 201f
   circumscribed choroidal, 200, 201f, 295t
   juxtamedullary capillary, 184
   optic disc, 184
   retinal capillary, 184–185, 185f
   retinal cavernous, 186, 187f, 295t
Hemorrhage
   blot, in nonproliferative diabetic retinopathy, 56
   flame-shaped, in nonproliferative diabetic retinopathy, 56
   intraretinal, in nonproliferative diabetic retinopathy, 56, 56f

premacular, 144, 145f
in retinal artery macroaneurysm, 102
salmon patch, in sickle cell retinopathy, 106
submacular, 17–19, 18f
subretinal, and angioid streaks, 40, 41f, 42, 43f
vitreous, in proliferative diabetic retinopathy, 66, 67f, 68f, 69f, 72f
Heredopathia atactica polyneuritiformis. See Refsum's disease
Hermansky-Pudlak syndrome, and albinism, 166, 167f
Highly active antiretroviral therapy (HAART), 118
Histoplasma capsulatum, and presumed ocular histoplasmosis syndrome, 127
HIV. See Human immunodeficiency virus
Hollenhorst plaque
   in branch retinal artery obstruction, 84
   in central retinal artery obstruction, 86, 87f
   in cilioretinal artery obstruction, 83
Homocystinuria, and dislocated lens, 250
Horseshoe (flap) tears of retina, 259, 259f, 262f, 263f, 274, 275f
Human immunodeficiency virus (HIV)
   and cytomegalovirus retinitis, 118, 119f
   retinopathy of, 125–126, 125f
   and syphilitic chorioretinitis, 123
Hydroxychloroquine retinopathy, 254
HYE. See Hard yellow exudates
Hyperplasia, reactive, of retinal pigment epithelium, 295t
Hypertension, and cotton-wool spots, 77
Hypertensive choroidopathy, 78
Hypertensive retinopathy, 78–81, 79f, 80f
Hypertrophy, congenital, of retinal pigment epithelium, 188, 189f, 295t
Hypoplasia, foveal, 289t
Hypotony maculopathy, 52, 53f

ICROP. See International Classification of Retinopathy of Prematurity
Idiopathic macular hole, 26–28, 26t, 27f, 28f, 29f

Stickler's syndrome, 274, 275*f*
Strabismus, and retinoblastoma, 180, 181*f*
Streptococcus
  and acute postoperative endophthalmitis, 114, 115
  and bleb-associated endophthalmitis, 116
Stretch tears of retina, 259, 260*f*
Submacular hemorrhage, 17–19, 18*f*
Subretinal hemorrhage, and angioid streaks, 40, 41*f*, 42, 42*f*, 43*f*
Sulfadiazine, for ocular toxoplasmosis, 117
Surface wrinkling retinopathy. *See* Macular epiretinal membrane
Sympathetic ophthalmia, 134–135, 135*f*
Sympathizing eye, in sympathetic ophthalmia, 134
Syphilitic chorioretinitis, 122–123, 123*f*

Talc retinopathy, 252, 253*f*, 253*t*
Tamoxifen (Nolvadex), and talc retinopathy, 252
Telangiectasia
  localized, 218*t*
  parafoveal, 104–105, 105*f*, 218*t*
  retinal. *See* Coats' disease
Teletherapy, and radiation retinopathy, 108, 109*f*
Temporary balloon, for rhegmatogenous retinal detachment, 268
Terson's syndrome, 240, 241*f*
Tetracyclines, second-generation, for ocular toxoplasmosis, 117
Thermal laser coagulation, for exudative age-related macular degeneration, 19, 20*f*
Thiabendazole, for diffuse unilateral subacute neuroretinitis, 127
Thioridazine retinopathy, 256, 257*f*
Threshold disease, of retinopathy of prematurity, 206, 209*f*
Tobramycin, for acute postoperative endophthalmitis, 115
Toxic retinopathies, 228–256
Toxocara canis, 117
  and diffuse unilateral subacute neuroretinitis, 126

Toxocariasis, ocular, 117–118
Toxoplasma gondii, 116
Toxoplasmosis, ocular, 19*f*, 116–117
Toxoplasmosis chorioretinitis, 116–117, 117*f*
Trauma, angioid streaks and, 42, 43*f*
Traumatic endophthalmitis, 116
Traumatic macular hole, 244, 245*f*
Traumatic retinopathies, 228–256
Treponema pallidum, 122–123
Trimethoprim-sulfamethoxazole, for ocular toxoplasmosis, 117
True albinism, 164
TS. *See* Tuberous sclerosis
Tuberous sclerosis (TS), and astrocytic hamartomas, 178–179
Tumors
  choroidal, 178–204
  retinal, 178–204
Type A personality, and central serous retinopathy, 44

Usher's syndrome, 172

Valsalva retinopathy, 216, 217*f*
Vancomycin, for acute postoperative endophthalmitis, 115
Vasculitis, retinal, 289*t*
Vasculopathy, polypoidal choroidal, 19
Venous beading, in nonproliferative diabetic retinopathy, 56, 58*f*
Verteporfin photodynamic therapy
  for degenerative myopia, 39
  for exudative age-related macular degeneration, 19, 20*f*, 21*f*
Vitamin A
  for Bassen-Kornzweig syndrome, 172
  for retinitis pigmentosa, 171
Vitamin B_6, for gyrate atrophy, 161
Vitamin E, for Bassen-Kornzweig syndrome, 172
Vitelliform disease, 297*t*
Vitelliform stage, of Best's disease, 142, 143*f*
Vitelliruptive stage, of Best's disease, 144, 145*f*

Vitrectomy
  for endophthalmitis, 115*t*
  for proliferative diabetic retinopathy, 70, 72*f*, 73*f*
  for rhegmatogenous retinal detachment, 269
Vitreomacular traction syndrome, 30–31, 31*f*
Vitreoretinal tuft, 276, 277*f*
Vitreoretinopathy
  familial exudative, 214, 215*f*, 297*t*
  proliferative, 270–271, 270*t*, 271*f*, 272*f*, 273*f*

Vitreous base, avulsed, 232, 233*f*
Vitreous hemorrhage, in proliferative diabetic retinopathy, 66, 67*f*, 68*f*, 69*f*, 72*f*
VKH. *See* Vogt-Koyanagi-Harada syndrome
Vogt-Koyanagi-Harada (VKH) syndrome, 133–134, 133*f*, 133*t*
Von Hippel-Lindau syndrome, 184

Weill-Marchesani syndrome, and dislocated lens, 250